Diseases of
Domestic Rabbits

LIBRARY OF VETERINARY PRACTICE

LIBRARY OF VETERINARY PRACTICE

Diseases of
Domestic Rabbits

LIEVE OKERMAN
Faculty of Veterinary Medicine
Casinoplein 24
B-9000 Gent
Belgium

TRANSLATED BY
RICHARD SUNDAHL

BLACKWELL SCIENTIFIC PUBLICATIONS

OXFORD LONDON EDINBURGH

BOSTON PALO ALTO MELBOURNE

© 1988 by
Blackwell Scientific Publications
Editorial offices:
Osney Mead, Oxford, OX2 0EL
(Orders: Tel. 0865 240201)
8 John Street, London WC1N 2ES
23 Ainslie Place, Edinburgh EH3 6AJ
3 Cambridge Center, Suite 208
   Cambridge, Massachusetts
   02142, USA
667 Lytton Avenue, Palo Alto
   California 94301, USA
107 Barry Street, Carlton
   Victoria 3053, Australia

First published 1988

Set by Times Graphics, Singapore
Printed and bound in Great Britain
by Billing & Sons Ltd,
Worcester

DISTRIBUTORS

USA
   Year Book Medical Publishers
   200 North LaSalle Street,
   Chicago, Illinois 60601
   (Orders: Tel. 312 726-9733)

Canada
   The C.V. Mosby Company
   5240 Finch Avenue East
   Scarborough, Ontario
   (Orders: Tel. 416-298-1588)

Australia
   Blackwell Scientific Publications
   (Australia) Pty Ltd
   107 Barry Street
   Carlton, Victoria 3053
   (Orders: Tel. (03) 347 0300)

British Library
Cataloguing in Publication Data

Okerman, Lieve
   Diseases of domestic rabbits.
   1. Livestock. Rabbits. Diseases
   I. Title   II. Series
   636'.9322

ISBN 0-632-02254-X

Contents

Preface, vii

Part I: General and Zootechnical Background

1 Introduction, 3

2 General background, 4

3 Anatomical peculiarities, 9

4 Brief remarks on physiology, 13

5 Feeding, 15

6 Housing and hygiene, 18

7 Breeding and raising, 21

8 Behaviour, 23

Part II: Diseases and their Treatment

9 Handling for clinical examination and treatment, 27

10 Examination of the living animal, 29

11 Necropsy, 32

12 Microscopic and bacteriological examination as a
    diagnostic aid, 37

13 Diseases of the skin, 40

14 Diseases of the eye, 51

15 Diseases of the respiratory system, 53

16 Diseases of the digestive system, 58

17 Diseases of the urogenital system, 75

18 Disorders of the nervous system and related conditions, 78

19 Systemic diseases, 81

20 Inherited conditions, 86

21 Breeding problems, 90

22 Administration of medication, 97

23 Traumatology and surgical intervention: castration, 103

24 Anaesthesia and hypnosis, 105

25 Euthanasia, 110

26 Zoonotic aspects, 112

Bibliography and further reading, 114

Index, 117

Appendix: Most frequent problems with the different types of rabbit, *inside back cover*

Colour plates 1–28 appear between pages 72 and 73

Preface

This book was originally written in Dutch after I had acquired 8 years of experience working on a research project entitled *Etiology and Pathogenesis of Broiler Rabbit Diseases*, which was financially supported by a grant from the Instituut ter Bevordering van het Wetenschappelijk Onderzoek in Nijverheid en Landbouw (IWONL, Brussels, Belgium). The project was headed by Professor Albert Devos, formerly Chairman of the Poultry Pathology—Bacteriology—Infectious Diseases Department in the Faculty of Veterinary Medicine, University of Gent, and by the late Professor Leo Spanoghe. I gained practical experience in the clinic for birds, fur animals and exotic pets of the same department. Though this project came to an end in July 1984, I have continued with research on the same and related subjects on a voluntary basis. I am ever grateful to Professor A. Devos for his encouragement and for the departmental facilities put at my disposal.

Following a suggestion by Dr Gunindra N. Dutta, an Indian colleague and personal friend, the original text was translated into English by another good friend, Richard Sundahl, whose linguistic skills and sense for perfection I admire.

I wish to express my gratitude to a number of persons who have helped me in acquiring knowledge and experience of rabbit matters and/or by criticizing the manuscript. My father, Frans Okerman, formerly head of the Breeding and Genetics section at the State Institute for Small Stock Husbandry, Merelbeke, Belgium, is to be mentioned here first, because it was his love for small farm animals, and especially for rabbits, which inspired me to choose my profession in the same specialty. Also his help in writing the chapters on housing, breeding, genetics and feeding—subjects which have formed a major part of his work for many years—was greatly appreciated.

Other Belgian rabbit specialists have helped me a great deal, both through exchange of information and fruitful discussion. In particular, I wish to thank Luc Maertens (State Institute for Small Stock Husbandry, Merelbeke), Johan Peeters (National Institute for Veterinary Research, Brussels), and Lea Van den Broeck (President of the Belgian Branch of the World Rabbit Science Association).

My colleagues at the Faculty of Veterinary Medicine should also be acknowledged for their support, and especially those who helped with certain specialized chapters of the book. Frank Gasthuys provided much valuable information on anaesthesia; Paul Simoens assisted with the chapter on anatomy; Piet Van Bree is thanked for technical assistance; Chris Van den Hende was helpful with the section on clinical chemistry, and Professor Joseph Vercruysse updated the material on parasitic diseases.

Most of all, I want to thank one particular colleague, Luc Devriese, who also happens to be my husband. It goes without saying that without his moral support and scientific and editorial advice, as well as his help in the household, I would never have been able to finish this book.

Gent   L. OKERMAN
March 1988

Part I
General and Zootechnical
Background

1 / Introduction

Rabbits are raised for a variety of purposes, including their use in the laboratory. In Europe especially, they are raised for meat. Besides being efficient converters of vegetable protein into high-quality animal protein, they . . . breed like rabbits. Theoretically a doe is capable of producing 80 young per year, though in practice such a figure is attained only in rare cases. The fur constitutes a valuable by-product. Other uses include wool production; Angoras can produce up to 1000 grams of high quality wool per year. Moreover, purebred show animals are raised as a hobby, and rabbits of all shapes and colours are kept as pets.

The production of rabbit meat on an industrial scale has been very slow to develop, even in countries where the demand is great. The cause is technical rather than economic. Excessive mortality among the growing broiler rabbits and fertility problems among the does have hindered the transition to mass production.

Obviously the pathology of the rabbit differs greatly according to the type and use of the animal (pet, laboratory, 'backyard' or industrial). The author takes this fact into account and, when necessary, indicates in which type a given disease most commonly occurs.

The text is not intended as an exhaustive description of all diseases that occur in rabbits, but rather as an aid to veterinarians who in the course of their practice are called upon to treat them. Various topics only indirectly related to disease, such as feeding and housing, are also discussed, along with certain special characteristics of the species.

2 / General background

History and taxonomy

The European rabbit, *Oryctolagus cuniculus*, belongs together with the hares (genus *Lepus*) and the American cottontail rabbits (genus *Sylvilagus*) to the order *Lagomorpha*, family *Leporidae*. These are often wrongly classified as 'rodents'. The term 'rodents' is synonymous with *Rodentia*, which in fact refers to such animals as rats, mice and hamsters.

The natural territory of *Oryctolagus cuniculus* is limited to the European continent and North Africa. The species has been released, however, in many other regions of the world. In Britain it was introduced in the early Middle Ages, but did not occur in high numbers until the 19th century. In Australia and New Zealand, where they found an ideal climate and an absence of natural enemies, rabbits multiplied so rapidly as to become a veritable plague. The species has never managed to establish itself in North America, with the exception of some islands where feral rabbits (a reversion of the domesticated form) have settled. In South America wild *Oryctolagus* are only found in Chile.

Before the Christian era wild rabbits were abundant around the Mediterranean Basin. The word Spain may be a bastard form of the Phoenician name for the peninsula, which meant literally, 'land of the rabbits'. The Romans started keeping rabbits and hares within walled-in areas, the so-called 'leporaria' (which can be compared to the rabbit warrens that were used in Britain in the Middle Ages). Although the hares failed to reproduce under these conditions, the rabbits thrived and this is regarded by many as a beginning of domestication. True domestication, with housing in hutches, began late in the Middle Ages in the abbeys. In those days the unborn young were considered a delicacy. It proved to be more economical, though, to keep the does alive and slaughter the young just after birth, so the animals had to be kept in hutches. Production for meat in hutches did not begin until the last century and was a result of the Industrial Revolution. Farm workers had little area available for their own use, and factory workers even less. Rabbits require minimal space and relatively little food. Large-scale production did not appear until the

4

1960s, principally in France, Spain, Italy, Belgium, Holland, Britain and the Eastern European countries.

In the course of domestication, numerous mutations have created a great variety of sizes, fur colour and texture, colour of the iris, and so on. Readers with further interest in this topic will find more specialized literature in the selected bibliography at the end of this book.

Breeds

The largest rabbit breed, the Flemish Giant, sometimes grows to a weight of more than 9 kg, while the smallest, the Polish rabbit, barely reaches even 1 kg. Only those breeds of heavier medium weight, (4 to 5.5 kg adult weight) come into consideration for meat production.

The New Zealand White is well suited for meat production. This breed is also widely used as a laboratory animal. The Californian is white with dark-coloured extremities, that is, the nose, ears, paws and tail. Both these breeds have thick skin and sturdy paws, which makes them suitable for housing on wire floors.

Many regions have local breeds which produce high-quality meat and are very fertile, but they are usually less suited for breeding in batteries. The Burgundi Red, the Argenté de Champagne and the Dendermonde White belong to this type. These, along with all sorts of cross-breeds, are widely used in small-scale production.

On large farms selected strains and hybrids are used, in addition to the above-mentioned breeds. Hybrid rabbits ensure higher yields: more young, good milk production and rapid growth. On the other hand they cost more and, from a point of view of disease prevention, they have great disadvantages because the ongoing purchase of new stock brings with it the risk of disease.

Terminology

A female rabbit is called a doe or dam; a male is called a buck. New-born young are sometimes referred to as kits.

The size of an industrial rabbit farm is expressed in terms of the number of breeding cages, which is considered as a production unit; in France the term 'maternity cage' (*cage maternité*) is common. The number of maternity cages corresponds to the maximum number of does that can be in production at any particular time.

Since the yearly replacement percentage is often higher than 100%, the number of does that actually have been present on a farm in any given year will be higher than the number of maternity cages. Thus both investment and production (expressed in numbers of weaned young, total weight of slaughter rabbits, or financial yield) are calculated per maternity cage as a production unit. In Angora rabbit farms, however, the total number of animals present is taken into consideration.

Functional uses of the rabbit

Meat production

Advantages

Rabbits offer some advantages over other herbivores (cattle, sheep, horses) and omnivores (chickens, pigs):
1 In low-intensity raising the rabbit does not compete with man for its nutritional needs and it requires very little space. This is important for meat production in developing countries and during periods of crisis; during World Wars I and II large numbers of rabbits were raised on grass and kitchen waste in West European cities.
2 A doe is theoretically capable of producing several times its weight in young per year. When a litter is weaned at 5 weeks, its total weight often exceeds that of the mother. A doe should be capable of turning out about eight litters per year.
3 Rabbits produce a type of meat that is currently 'in'. It is higher in protein and water, and lower in fat, than that of other mammalian meat producers.

Disadvantages

1 Breeding animals must be individually housed. This means that the industrial rabbit farm is labour-intensive, at least when compared to large-scale poultry farming.
2 Broiler rabbits are extremely sensitive to diseases of the digestive tract. This is due to the special physiology of their digestion and to the fact that not very much research has yet been done on these disorders. Because of these disorders and because of fertility problems, the theoretically possible figure of 80 slaughter rabbits per doe is never

attained, or only occasionally by an individual animal. Actual production ranges from 30 to 50 young brought to slaughter per maternity cage.

Some guidelines for industrial rabbit production

1 Homogenous batches of animals are preferable because they bring a better wholesale price from the butcher; this homogeneity is attained by standardizing the size of the litters. The excess young in large litters are placed with foster does.
2 A higher percentage weight yield after slaughter also brings a higher price from the butcher. This percentage yield is genetically determined and varies according to the breed, but can be affected by the nutrition. Rabbits raised in battery cages and fed only pellets have a less developed digestive tract, and thus a lower percentage loss when butchered.

Wool production

Angora rabbits are excellent wool producers, yielding more wool per kilo body weight than sheep; namely 0.2 kg per kg body weight and per year. This wool is of very high quality and possesses a high insulation capacity. Females produce more and better wool than males.

On the other hand, raising Angoras for wool is labour-intensive, especially when they are hand-plucked. In Holland and Germany the animal protection laws require that they be shorn, even though the quality of shorn wool is lower than that of plucked. Shorn wool is used in the textile industry. Hand-plucked wool is very expensive and is sold for knitting. Both purposes have also led to differences in hair structure of the breeds: Angoras which are suitable for plucking cannot be shaved, or else the quality of the new wool will be bad. Angora rabbits which are kept as pets should be shorn with a hair clipper at regular intervals, otherwise they develop hair knots, and their fur will mat.

The rabbit as a laboratory animal

Because of its high fertility, short generation span, small size and low cost of maintenance the rabbit is an ideal laboratory animal, though many objections can be made against painful or unnecessary uses of these animals as laboratory tools.

Some applications

1 Teratological experiments: the moment of fertilization can always be known precisely because ovulation is induced by copulation. Moreover, there is close contact between maternal and fetal circulatory systems, as is also the case with human beings.
2 Suppliers of tissue cultures.
3 Toxicity tests; detection of pyrogens.
4 Ophthalmology.

By preference, SPF (specific pathogen free) animals are used. As these are not readily available and rather expensive, ordinary animals can be bought and kept in quarantine for a certain period.

3 / Anatomical peculiarities

External

The mouth opening is small, so that a thorough examination of the mouth cavity is impossible.

Some breeds have a fold of skin in the throat area which is called the dewlap. The dewlap is most pronounced in older does. This should not be mistaken as an abnormal growth or even an abscess (see Plate 1).

Skeleton and muscles

In countries where rabbit meat is a common part of the diet, concerned consumers regularly show up at the veterinarian's office with a headless rabbit carcass that, almost always mistakenly, they suspect to be a cat. The colour of the raw meat clearly distinguishes the two: cat meat is dark red, while that of domesticated rabbit is light pink. The most obvious skeletal differences are cited in Table 3.1 and Fig. 3.1.

Digestive system

Dental formula: I (2/1); C (0/0); PM (3/2); M (3/3).

The two upper incisors are situated not beside but behind each other. The front uppers and lowers are continually growing and wearing each other down. The backmost upper incisors are called peg teeth.

The stomach is large and thin-walled. The relatively flat and long spleen (2–4 cm long) lies attached to the stomach. The duodenum is relatively long. The pancreas is diffuse and difficult to locate in the fatty tissue. The most prominent organ is the very large caecum. The ileum ends in the caecum as a thickening called the sacculus rotundus. The corpus caeci is large and thin-walled and ends in a thick-walled appendix. Lymphoid tissue is concentrated in the Peyer's patches, the sacculus rotundus and the appendix. The caecum runs gradually into the colon. Two anal glands have

9

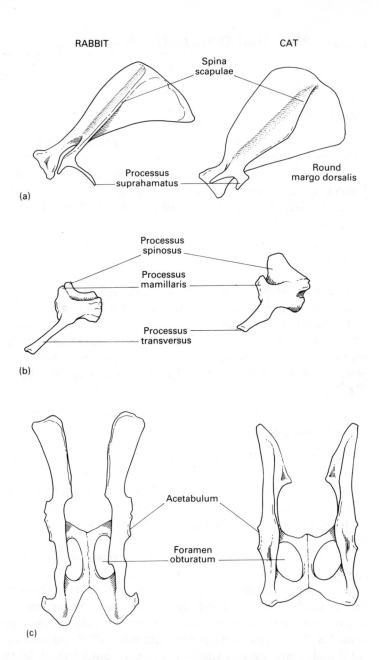

Fig. 3.1. The most important skeletal differences between rabbits and cats. (a) Scapula; (b) fourth lumbar vertebra; (c) pelvis (dorsal view).

Table 3.1 Most obvious skeletal differences between the rabbit and the cat

Rabbit	Cat
Scapula (Fig. 3.1)	
Triangular	Rounded margo dorsalis
Length greater than breadth	Equal breadth and length
Spina located $\frac{1}{4}$ to $\frac{1}{3}$ of distance from cranial edge	Spina located more or less in the middle
Acromion deeply recessed with long processus suprahamatus	Acromion not deeply recessed with short processus suprahamatus
Fore-limb	
Radius and ulna are fused and clearly bowed (fusion is only complete in older animals)	Radius and ulna are separate and straight
Ribs	
Flattened	More rounded
Lumbar vertebrae (Fig. 3.1)	
Processus mamillaris about equally as long as processus spinosus	Processus mamillaris half as long as processus spinosus
Processus transversus long and narrow	Processus transversus broad
Pelvis (Fig. 3.1)	
Ratio length : breadth >2 : 1	Ratio length : breadth <2 : 1
Foramen obturatum is clearly oval	Foramen obturatum is practically round
Acetabulum half-way between front and back edge	Acetabulum further from front than from back edge
Leg	
The fibula is developed over only half the length of the tibia and is fused with it	The fully developed fibula is not fused with the tibia

openings into the rectum. See Fig. 3.2 for a schematic drawing of the digestive system.

Urogenital system

The uterus has two horns and two separate cervices. The placenta is of the haemochorial type. Because of this, the maternal and fetal circulatory systems are in very close contact (as with human beings).

In males the testicles descend at around 3 months, and before this age castration is difficult or even impossible. The testicles can be retracted into the abdominal cavity.

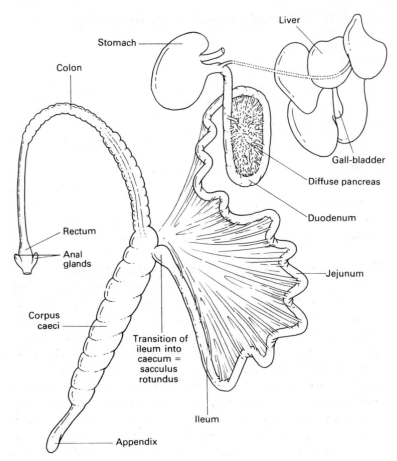

Fig. 3.2. Schematic drawing of the intestinal tract.

Sex determination before the age of 2 months is difficult, and even experienced raisers sometimes make a mistake. In young females the urinary opening takes the form of a split, while in males it is round. With older males the penis can be made to appear by lightly pressing, but this is not possible with younger rabbits. Of course once the testicles descend there is no longer any doubt.

4 / Brief remarks on physiology

Body temperature: 39.5°C.
Pulse: about 300 per minute.
Breath rate: 32–60 per minute.
Oestrus cycle: mating induces ovulation. See below, Chapter 7: breeding and raising.
Duration of pregnancy: average 31–32 days.
Litter size: 1–12 young, sometimes more, depending on the breed. Small breeds have small litters.
Life expectancy: 7–8 years. Breeding does are reproductive for 2–3 years.

The digestive physiology of the rabbit is quite unusual compared with that of other domestic animals. This is due to the phenomenon called caecotrophy. Caecotrophy is a more appropriate name than coprophagy; the term reingestion may also be used. In the uncommonly large caecum of the rabbit a process takes place that is more or less comparable with the digestion in the first stomach of the ruminants: the transformation of vegetable protein into high-quality bacterial protein and the digestion of raw fibre. In the beginning of the colon a differentiation is made between two sorts of droppings: the 'hard droppings', which are rich in fibres and are simply eliminated, and the 'soft droppings' or caecotrophs, which are richer in water and micro-organisms. These caecotrophs are eliminated in 2- or 3-cm long packets which are immediately ingested directly from the anus. At necropsy the caecotrophs can be found in the fundus section of the stomach. Only rarely can they be found on the bottom of the cage.

Randomly fed rabbits follow a definite 24-hour rhythm in their eating habits. Feeding takes place primarily in the evening, night and early morning. The hard droppings are eliminated at the same time. Caecotrophy takes place during the day (between 9 a.m. and 5 p.m.).

The concentration of volatile fatty acids in the serum is very high, just as with the ruminants. Absorption takes place primarily in the caecum and to a lesser degree in the colon, but not in the stomach, even though the caecotrophs remain there for a period of time.

The caecotrophy process is controlled by the adrenal glands. It is

13

Table 4.1 Haematological values

Constituent	Unit	Range
Haemoglobin	g %	10.9–14.5
Packed cell volume	%	31–40
Red blood cells	$\times 10^6/cm^3$	3.9–5.8
White blood cells	$\times 10^3/cm^3$	2.5–7.5
Total protein	g/100 ml	5.4–7.4
Albumin	%	55
• α-globulin	%	15
• β-globulin	%	15
• γ-globulin	%	15
Sedimentation rate	cm/24 h	0.5–2
Bilirubin	$u$mol/l	3–7
Urea	mmol/l	7–13
Calcium	mmol/l	2.4–3.4
Magnesium	mmol/l	0.5–0.8
Sodium	mmol/l	128–148
Potassium	mmol/l	3.3–4.1
Alkaline phosphatase	iu/l	10–50
SGOT	iu/l	10–30
SGPT	iu/l	10–30
Glucose	mmol/l	3–8

generally supposed that stress situations hinder the formation of the caecotrophs and thus have a negative effect on digestion.

As for the microflora, one peculiarity should be noted, namely the almost total absence of *Escherichia coli* in the caecal contents of healthy weaned rabbits. Suckling rabbits of 2–3 weeks of age have a temporary high *E. coli* count in the caecum contents. In weaned animals, the intestinal flora consists almost exclusively of Gram-negative strict anaerobes (*Bacteroides* spp.). The cause of this is probably the inhibiting effect of the volatile fatty acids, together with the slightly acid pH environment of the caecal contents. If the pH level rises as a result of some digestive disorder (coccidiosis, for example), then the inhibiting effect diminishes and *E. coli* nevertheless will appear. Thus a raised *E. coli* count ($>10^3$/g of caecal contents) does not necessarily indicate coli-diarrhoea.

Few blood and urine tests have been adapted for use with rabbits. In appearance the urine is cloudy, and microscopic examination of the sediment shows that it consists of amorphous crystals. The pH is about 8.2. Some blood values can be found in Table 4.1.

5 / Feeding

General facts

- Daily feed consumption (dry rabbit pellets): about 5% of body weight.
- Feed conversion: optimally 3:1.
- Daily water consumption: about 10% of body weight.
Exception: lactating does consume much more feed and water. The total water consumption depends on the number of young and on the time in the lactation period. It often amounts to more than 1 litre per day. Maximum milk production occurs at around 3 weeks post-partum.
- Rabbits can be very choosy and refuse feed other than the type they are used to. Also, when new batches of pellets are given, food intake may be lower for a few days. Some animals may be so stubborn that they would eventually starve rather than try the new feed.

Feeding of rabbits in large-scale farms

In industrial situations, rabbits are always fed with commercially available pellets. This is the only suitable feed for such purposes. Rabbit pellets should be 3–5 mm thick and 1 cm long. For practical reasons nursing does and growing broiler rabbits are given the same feed, even though separate and different feeding could give better results. See Chapter 22, Table 22.2 for a table of approximate daily quantities of water and feed consumed.

The influence of the raw fibre content on the health of the animals can be summarized as follows. Cellulose remains for the greater part undigested and yet it is necessary as ballast for the healthy working of the intestines. The raw fibre must not be too finely ground. On the other hand, if the fibre is too coarse the pellets will easily break, so a happy medium must be found. When the raw cellulose content is too low, or when the fibre is too finely ground, the risk of diarrhoea is increased because of the slowed passage through the intestines. This fact is very often confirmed in practice, and yet laboratory studies have shown that even though extremely low fibre content will slow growth, it will not increase mortality. It is also known that although optimal fibre content will reduce the frequency of digestive disorders, it will not eliminate them. The pathogenic agents seem to play a decisive role in this respect. More detailed information on this subject can be found in Chapter 16. Supplementing the diet with hay and straw is good for the functioning of the intestines, but has a negative effect on growth and feed conversion. This practice is also difficult in industrial situations because it often blocks the manure-removal system. Another advantage of hay and straw is its preventive effect on fur plucking by hutchmates and on trichobezoars in adults.

Feed rationing

Feed is seldom rationed; this practice increases the work hours, as feeding must occur daily and at a regular time. Besides this, broiler rabbits and does in late pregnancy and while nursing should not be rationed since this lowers their productivity. On the other hand, does that are immature, not yet pregnant, or in the first half of pregnancy, and also bucks may be rationed. Rationing of broiler rabbits has a favourable effect in the prevention of certain digestive disorders, especially mucoid enteropathy.

Poisoning

Like ducks, rabbits are very sensitive to aflatoxins. Therefore certain feed ingredients, such as groundnut by-products, should be avoided. Other ingredients such as alfalfa and corn can also contain aflatoxins. Experiments have shown that rabbits usually refuse mouldy feed, so in practice aflatoxicosis and other mycotoxicoses are not a problem in rabbits.

Toxic plants, such as foxgloves and many others, are not usually eaten by rabbits. An exception is a weed called woolly-pod milkweed, which grows in the Pacific South-West of the United States and which produces paralysis and death.

Plants containing tropine esters such as belladonna leaves can be eaten by some rabbits that have an enzyme known as serum atropinesterase in their serum. This faculty is controlled by a semidominant gene. It should be noted here that the presence or absence of this enzyme also determines how the animal will respond to atropine, if it is given by injection or administered topically to the eye.

Pet rabbits can be poisoned by exotic house and garden plants, such as Dieffenbachia and Cytisus.

Feeding of 'backyard' and show rabbits

Pellet feeding has also become common with these types of rabbits, although the diet is usually supplemented with hay, greens, beets, bread and kitchen waste. Coccidiosis appears very often in such groups because the animals receive too little of the coccidiostat which is always incorporated in commercial pellets. Group treatment is also a problem. Whenever the feed has a high moisture content (for example, greens) the rabbits drink very little or no water, in which case the medication obviously cannot be administered via the drinking water.

There are still other disadvantages of supplemental feeding with greens:
1 The risk of parasitic diseases such as toxoplasmosis, cysticercosis, nematode infestations and hepatic distomiasis increases.
2 Growth is retarded.

These arguments fail, however, to convince most small-scale raisers, not only because the supplemental feed is so much cheaper, but also because they claim it gives the meat a better flavour.

Feeding of pet rabbits

Hamster and mouse pellets that are available in retail outlets are not suitable for rabbits. Guinea-pig feed is suitable for rabbits, although the converse is not true, since guinea-pigs must have vitamin C in their diet (note: guinea-pig feed that is several months old also no longer contains sufficient vitamin C). The rabbit pellets sold in small packages are relatively expensive. It is usually cheaper to feed pet rabbits with bread, pieces of fruit and vegetable waste. Oats, barley and hay are very good supplements.

A weaned rabbit should be given only water to drink, not milk. Some rabbits drink little or no water, especially when they are given a lot of greens. Nevertheless, a bowl of fresh water should always be available.

6 / Housing and hygiene

Does are housed individually. For smaller numbers wooden or concrete hutches are used, with straw on the floor. Wooden hutches are covered on the inside with plating so that the animals cannot gnaw through them. A slightly sloping floor helps keep the floor-covering dry, which is important for the prevention of coccidiosis. The usual dimensions are 80 cm broad × 60 cm deep × 50 cm high. A separate nest space is sometimes provided. When the animals are housed individually the litter needs to be replaced only once a month, though fresh straw should be added regularly.

These hutches are placed in an unheated shed or under an overhanging roof in a protected location. Adult rabbits can tolerate very low temperatures as long as they are kept dry and out of draughts.

Angora rabbits are housed in these traditional hutches, since wire cages are not suitable for them. The hutches should be relatively large, because otherwise the animals cannot keep their fur clean. As cold temperatures favour wool formation the sheds are not heated in wintertime. An infra-red lamp must be placed in the hutches during the first 24–48 hours after the rabbits have been plucked or shorn.

Large-scale production of rabbits requires the use of battery cages with wire mesh flooring, both for broilers and breeding stock. A wire mesh suitable for rabbits should be used, and even then not all breeds can tolerate it (see sections on sore hocks in Chapters 13 and 19). Plastic grilles are sometimes used for adult bucks and does. These are less traumatic for the paws and still acceptable from a hygienic point of view.

Broiler rabbits are housed separately from the does while being fattened. They are usually kept in small groups (four to eight per cage).

As for the does, a nest space must always be provided shortly before littering. The current practice is to install a nest box on the outside of the cage. This need not be any larger than 30 × 30 cm in floor area. A doe prefers a dark nest box with a floor lower than that of the rest of the hutch. These boxes are constructed of wood, metal or synthetic materials. Some have a wire mesh floor. If the mesh is too large, a perforated board can be laid on top of it. Some material

18

suitable for nest building, usually straw or wood shavings, is provided shortly before the doe is due to give birth.

In the northern latitudes (especially continental Europe) these wire cages are set up in closed sheds with heating in the winter. The ideal temperature is 15°C. Lower temperatures increase feed consumption; very low temperatures inhibit production because of mortality in the nest.

It is possible, however, to set up wire cages in the open, with only a corrugated roof to cover them, as is common in England. In the winter the sides are covered with plastic sheeting. Another cheap method of housing is the so-called 'rabbit tunnel', which is constructed of plastic sheeting on a metal frame and provides only minimal protection against changes in the weather.

Both types of sheds are used in all, including northern, climatic conditions. Despite temperature extremes, the rabbits thrive. The breed used in England has been selected for its resistance to cold. In addition, the nest boxes are made larger and in winter-time are provided with a thick layer of straw and wood shavings. Even though the production per individual animal is lower with this system, the net production is good because of the lower initial building investment and the lack of ongoing costs for lighting, heating and ventilation.

Both the batteries for fattening young fryers and those for breeding can be of flat-deck construction. They can also be either staircase or multi-level in design. For manure removal there are several different systems in use, including: (a) the central trough with automatic flushing; (b) a system with conveyor belts; (c) the 'deep well' system in which the manure collects for several months in a 1-2 metre-deep well underneath the batteries.

Keeping a large distance between the accumulating manure and the mesh floors of the hutches is important for the prevention of coccidiosis. The worst system in this respect is that with collecting pans or conveyor belts running immediately under the mesh floors in multi-level batteries.

Hygienic measures which should be practised in all large-scale rabbitries

Wool and hair left clinging to the cages can only be removed with a gas burner. When the rabbits are infected with dermatophytes this wool must be regularly removed. Obviously the cages have to be constructed of materials which can resist this treatment.

The all-in, all-out system can only be used in operations with well-separated compartments. Disinfection can never be 100% when this is not the case since there are always living animals within the enclosure. In any case certain measures are absolutely necessary in all types of rabbitries:

1 Disinfection of the nest box whenever a litter is weaned, especially when the box is to be transferred to another doe.

2 Disinfection of the hutch when a doe is eliminated and a new doe is to be placed in it.

3 Disinfection of the cages after removal of a batch of fryers.

Separately removable cages are thus preferable, even though more expensive.

7 / Breeding and raising

In industrial rabbitries the does are first mated when they are around 4 months old. Heavier breeds mature later, lighter breeds earlier. This is also true of the bucks which, in the case of smaller breeds, are sometimes active at 3 months. In general the males are left 1 month longer than does before being bred. Breeders of show rabbits wait even longer to start breeding.

The young are born 29–32 days later, but in most cases after 31 or 32 days. Litter size varies from one to twelve, seldom more. They are nursed once or sometimes twice a day. The eyes open around the tenth day. During the third week they start hopping about and are able to eat solid food. At 4 weeks they can be weaned.

With an intensive breeding rate the does are mated again immediately after giving birth. This requires that the young be weaned at the latest after 4 weeks.

When a semi intensive rhythm is followed the doe is again mated 10–12 days post-partum. The young are weaned at 4–6 weeks. This is the most usual system among European industrial raisers.

The extensive breeding rhythm is used for show and backyard rabbits and in the English open-air method (see Chapter 6). The doe is not mated again until the previous litter is at least 6 weeks old, i.e. at or after the time of weaning.

Artificial insemination is possible and relatively simple, although its practical application remains limited. Immediately before being inseminated, does must be given an intramuscular injection of 0.0008 mg buserelin, a synthetic releasing factor which sets the luteinizing and the follicle-stimulating hormones free. Without this, they will not ovulate.

Partus can be induced with 1–2 iu of oxytocin, administered by intramuscular injection.

The young rabbits reach slaughter weight at 10–12 weeks. Does to be used for breeding are housed separately after 3 months in order to avoid pseudopregnancy.

Pregnancy detection

An experienced handler can detect pregnancy in a doe that has been mated at least 10–12 days before, by palpation. The animal is placed on a rough table with the ears and skin of the neck held down by the left hand. The right hand is used to palpate the abdominal area just in front of the pelvis, being careful not to press too hard. Through the abdominal lining the fetuses can be felt between the fingertips. Palpation is safest between the tenth and fourteenth day; thereafter the risk of damage to the fetuses increases.

Another method, though less reliable, is to place the doe with the buck again. Pregnant does usually do not let themselves be mounted, but this is also too often the case with does that are not pregnant.

8 / Behaviour

Many peculiarities of behaviour among domesticated rabbits can be explained in terms of the psychology of their wild relatives. Wild rabbits live in groups (colonies) with a clear hierarchy among both bucks and does. The bucks each choose a permanent mate, and those higher in the hierarchy often also have one or more 'mistresses'. The tunnels are dug by pregnant females in order to build their nests. This explains the negative experiences of those who have attempted to raise rabbits in colonies with a ratio of approximately one buck for ten does: in the first place, the females that are preparing to give birth fight for the same nest space; furthermore, the buck chooses certain does and refuses to mount the others.

Behaviour of pet rabbits

1 *Cleanliness.* Rabbits generally have very clean habits and they always deposit their droppings and urine in the same place. Adult bucks, however, mark out their territory by rubbing their chins on certain landmarks. Glands that produce an odoriferous secretion are located under the chin, and are more developed in male rabbits. They also deposit strongly smelling droppings in scattered places for the same purpose.

2 *Tunnel digging.* This can be a problem with rabbits that run free in the garden. In order to prevent escape, the edge of the garden should be lined 30 cm deep with either concrete plates or wire mesh. It is only the females that dig the very deep tunnels, when they are pregnant or pseudo-pregnant.

3 *Taming* rabbits usually poses no problem. Most rabbits never attack or bite, but there are exceptions. Some breeds are easier in this respect than others, and there are great individual differences. Dwarf rabbits are nervous and sometimes aggressive. French lops are calm and languid and usually permit themselves to be handled. Wild *Oryctolagus* and crosses of wild and domestic breeds are impossible to tame; it is almost impossible even to keep them in an enclosed area.

4 *Housing.* Domestic rabbits can be kept together in the same space with all sorts of different animals (for example, dogs) as long as the

other animals adapt themselves to the rabbits. Cohabitation with guinea pigs is never a problem. Two rabbits in one cage, however, may create problems. Fighting can result in mutilation, especially of head and ears, and also castration of males which are mixed either with other males or with females. Preventive castration of males does not necessarily rule out fighting. Certain breeds, notably the New Zealand White, are much less aggressive towards their own kind than other breeds, but they can be aggressive to humans.

5 *Alarm signals.* When danger threatens, one wild rabbit will warn the others by loudly stamping its hind paws on the ground. This also happens with groups of caged rabbits, for example, when a strange person approaches: one after another, they all sound the alarm. A rabbit in deadly fear emits a penetrating cry; the others react by keeping still as a mouse. Rabbits with breathing difficulties (such as pneumonia) can also squeal in the same way.

6 *Pain.* Gnashing of the teeth is the typical expression of pain.

Part II
Diseases and their Treatment

9 / Handling for clinical examination and treatment

In order to lift it out of its cage or box, a rabbit is picked up by the loose skin of the neck, not by the ears or the legs. At the same time the hind paws should also be supported, especially with heavy animals. Young rabbits can also be picked up by grasping the loin area, and keeping the head down. Watch out with nursing does and with some aggressive rabbits: they will attack the hand reaching for them and they can bite hard and fast (cf. *Monty Python and the Holy Grail*). Young rabbits are the most likely to resist being held; their hind paws can injure the hands and arms of the carrier.

When carrying the animal, its body must be supported in order to avoid trauma to the spine. For a right-handed individual the best method is to hold the rabbit against the body with the head to the carrier's left. With the right hand the skin of the neck is held fast and the rabbit is pressed against the body. With the left hand the hind feet are held together while the left arm supports the body from underneath.

For examination or for treatment, the animal is placed on a table. A rabbit panics when placed on a smooth surface, so many rabbit raisers nail a gunny sack on an old table. If this is not available, a heavy floor mat or some such thing can be used with a nervous animal.

To immobilize the animal, a number of different designs are available for boxes or fixation cages which the raiser him/herself can construct. These are often used in laboratories. An experienced helper, however, is more effective than any of these other aids.

A normal, calm rabbit will hardly react to subcutaneous injections, so neither a helper nor fixation is necessary. The injection is given in the loose skin of the back, preferably between the shoulderblades. This is especially important for vaccinations because a local vaccinal reaction in this area makes for the least problems.

A helper is needed for drawing blood and for giving intravenous or intramuscular injections. The helper holds the rabbit fast by the skin of the neck and of the lower back and then presses the animal firmly against the table.

For drawing blood and for intravenous injections the marginal ear vein is most often used. The middle ear vein is larger but more difficult because it is less well fixed. Xylol is applied on the auricle, to dilate the veins. This substance is an irritant which causes immediate vasodilatation. It cannot be used when a white blood cell count is to be taken. The xylol is immediately wiped off with a dry piece of gauze. Note: xylol attacks plastics. After about 1 minute the ear vein becomes sufficiently dilated. The needle is positioned about one-third of the way down from the top of the ear. If the first attempt fails, a second can be made more proximally for intravenous injections, and more distally for blood drawing.

To draw blood, a 23 gauge injection needle is used to puncture the ear vein and immediately removed. The dripping or slowly flowing blood is caught in a test tube. When sufficient blood has been collected, pressure is applied directly to the puncture with a piece of gauze and is maintained until the bleeding stops. If necessary, a haemostatic product can be used. Collecting 5 ml of blood with this method is no problem. After drawing the blood the remainder of the xylol should be removed by washing with alcohol and water. Cardiac puncture is used for sterile blood drawing or when larger quantities are needed. This method is employed only in the laboratory and on anaesthesized animals; for details, see Chapter 25. Other methods are available, but they are more complicated.

For intravenous injections the same technique is employed. It should be noted here that xylol will not cause dilatation of the ear veins when the rabbit is in a state of shock. If necessary, the tarsal vein or the vena cephalica can be used.

For intramuscular injections, the rabbit must be held fast by a helper. The injection can be placed in the thigh muscles or in the withers.

Intradermal injection is sometimes prescribed for myxomatosis vaccines. A special apparatus called a dermojet, which injects the substance under high pressure, can be used for this purpose.

10 / Examination of the living animal

In this chapter, frequently occurring symptoms, external lesions or other findings in rabbits that are presented at the veterinary surgery are summed up. The most probable origins of these problems are indicated. For more detailed information the appropriate chapters should be consulted.

Skin fold under the chin (Plate 1):
• This is normal. It is most pronounced with older does and called the dewlap. The skin in the deep fold can, however, be irritated or inflamed. It is also a predilection site for a condition called 'moist dermatitis'.

Shedding hair on the head:
• Dermatomycosis.
• Ear mange.
• Fur plucking by cage mates.

Shedding hair on the back:
• Fur plucking by cage mates.
• Fur mites.

Shedding hair on breast and around teats:
• Nest building.

Skin infection:
• 'Moist dermatitis' = dermatitis caused by softening of the skin in areas that remain continuously moist.
• Staphylococcosis in very young animals.

Dirty in perineal region:
• Diarrhoea.
• Incontinence: fractured lumbar vertebrae.
• Pyometra in female animals.
• Abscesses in the anal glands.

Oedema of the head, most pronounced at the base of the ears:
• Myxomatosis.

Swellings:
• Myxomatosis.

- Abscesses.
- Malignant tumours are very rare, maybe because few rabbits grow old.

Crusts in earlobes:
- Ear mange.

Injuries of the sole of the foot:
- Ulcerative pododermatitis, also called 'sore hocks'.

Hairs sticking together on inside of front paws:
- Chronic snuffles or chronic conjunctivitis.

Dirty snout:
- Chronic snuffles, whether complicated or not.
- Pneumonia.
- Mucoid enteropathy–caecal-impaction complex.
- Irregularity of the molars causes hypersalivation.

Sneezing:
- Snuffles, pasteurellosis.

Respiratory noises (rattles):
- *Bordetella bronchiseptica* infection.

Dyspnoea:
- Enzootic pneumonia (pasteurellosis).
- Myxomatosis.

Diarrhoea:
- Hyperacute: enterotoxaemia.
- Acute to subacute: coli-enteritis, coccidiosis, Tyzzer's disease.

Weight loss without diarrhoea:
- Chronic sickness associated with weight loss.
- Dental abnormalities.
- Trichobezoars in the stomach.
- Rodentiosis.
- Coccidiosis.
- Other parasites.
- Sore hocks.
- Chronic form of Tyzzer's disease.

Straining:
- Urolithiasis
- Dystocia (rare).

Hind-limb paralysis:
- Coccidiosis.
- Trauma of the spine.
- Central nervous disorders of unknown origin.

Torticollis:
- Infection of the middle ear, due to *Pasteurella multocida*.
- Nosemosis.

Blindness:
- Inherited glaucoma.
- Disturbances of the central nervous system.
- Myxomatosis.

Note: Palpation of the abdomen can help to detect:
1 Trichobezoars in the stomach.
2 Caecal impaction-mucoid enteropathy: hard cord lower right in ventral region.
3 Pregnancy diagnosis (from twelfth day).
4 Tumours (very rare).
5 Pyometra (rather common).

11 / Necropsy

General

Before beginning the dissection, the nose and perineal region should be examined with special care, along with other aspects of the intact animal such as the body condition, ears, skin, etc. (see Chapter 10).

Post-mortem decay begins very quickly, especially when death occurs as a result of intestinal disorders. Bacteriological examination is almost useless with animals that have been dead for some time. *Pasteurella multocida* can no longer be recovered and many of the organs are flooded with bacteria that have swarmed post-mortem out of the intestinal system (*Escherichia coli*, *Proteus*). Only bacteria for which good selective media exist and which normally are not present (for example, *Salmonella*) can still be detected at this stage. Parasitological investigation is also still possible, except for the examination of direct organ smears when acute toxoplasmosis is suspected.

The aetiology of an intestinal disorder can only be properly investigated using a living, untreated animal that displays the typical symptoms. Histological examination of the intestines can be productive only when the organs are removed and fixed immediately after death. The same holds true for disorders of the nervous system when histological examination of the brain is necessary. Animals that have just died or just been destroyed are also needed for bacteriological interpretation of cultures for *E. coli*, and stainings for *Clostridium spiroforme* and *E. coli*.

Most common macroscopic lesions

Skin:
- See Chapter 10.
- Bite wounds.

Mouth cavity:
- Dental aberrations.

Nose cavity and sinuses:
- Presence of pus: snuffles, pasteurellosis. The head can be cleaved

32

lengthwise to give better access to these cavities. With young rabbits, this is very easily done. The cartilaginous septum can be removed with tweezers in order to obtain aseptically collected pus from the conchae.

Middle ear and bulla tympanica:
• The presence of pus should be investigated when signs of torticollis are present, and bacteriological examination for *Pasteurella multocida* is indicated.

Chest cavity:
• Haemorrhagic tracheitis: acute septicaemic pasteurellosis.
• Purulent to fibrinous (pleuro-) pneumonia and/or pericarditis: usually pasteurellosis.
• Lung abscesses: pasteurellosis or staphylococcosis.
• Hyperacute lung inflammation: septicaemic pasteurellosis.
• *Pseudomonas aeruginosa* infection.
• 'Foreign body' pneumonia (see section on Mucoid enteropathy, Chapter 16).
• Calcification of the large veins is occasionally seen in old rabbits.

Stomach:
• A few hours after death a layer of mucus forms on the wall of the stomach. This is a normal occurrence.
• Sometimes the stomach wall is torn. Usually this has happened post-mortem; if not, there should be haemorrhages and signs of inflammation in the area of the tear, as well as peritonitis.
• Nematodes: macroscopically visible as small, red worms on the inner surface of the stomach wall.
• Trichobezoars: principally in older rabbits and Angoras.
• Abnormal amount of water: caecal impaction — mucoid enteropathy.
• In healthy rabbits the stomach is never empty. In weaned animals it always contains fresh food and/or caecotrophs. In newborn rabbits, an empty stomach indicates agalactia of the mother.
• With rabbits which have died of diarrhoea, haemorrhages are sometimes seen on the stomach wall. The origin and significance are not clear.

Duodenum and jejunum:
• Gas formation and slight redness of the intestinal wall are normal in animals that have been dead for a few hours.

- Localized inflammation: coccidiosis, toxoplasmosis, unknown causes.
- Overfull:
1 Intestinal paresis in productives does.
2 Sometimes associated with mucoid enteropathy.

Ileum:
- Thickened intestinal wall: coccidiosis.

Sacculus rotundus:
- Necrotic foci: rodentiosis or salmonellosis.
- Narrowing of the passage leading from ileum to caecum: Tyzzer's disease.

Caecum:
- In a healthy rabbit the contents are soft and dark in colour. Upon cutting the caecum open, the contents do not spread out very far.
- All or parts of contents hard and dried up: caecal impaction — mucoid enteropathy complex.
- Oedema of the wall: Tyzzer's disease, coli-enteritis.
- Paintbrush haemorrhages: coli-enteritis, Tyzzer's disease.
- Severe haemorrhagic inflammation with or without actual haemorrhagic contents: coli-enteritis or enterotoxaemia.
- Fluid contents: coli-enteritis, intestinal paresis of does, coccidiosis, enterotoxaemia, unknown causes.
- Macroscopically visible small nematodes (sometimes in massive quantities): *Passalurus ambiguus*.

Appendix:
- Necrotic foci: rodentiosis or salmonellosis.

Colon:
- In the distal colon or rectum only well-formed droppings or caecotrophs are found in a healthy animal.
- Invagination is sometimes found with coli-enteritis.
- Lump of dried mucus: mucoid enteropathy.
- Gelatinous mass of mucus: intestinal paresis of does, mucoid enteropathy.
- The presence of mucus is possible with almost all intestinal infections.
- Fluid contents: the same causes as fluid contents in the caecum.

• Thin contents in the whole intestinal system, when accompanied by rawness of the visceral peritoneum and/or fibrinous or serous exudate in the peritoneal cavity: peritonitis.

Liver:
• Pea-sized abscesses: coccidiosis of the liver, often accompanied by macroscopically visible inflammation of the bile ducts. Bacterial causes are much more rare: *Escherichia coli* (mostly in baby rabbits), *Staphylococcus aureus, Salmonella*.
• Pinhead-sized foci:
1 Local: often found in normal, healthy animals when butchered.
2 Spread over the whole liver: Tyzzer's disease.
• Pale colour: excess fat (found commonly in older and fat does).
• Fibrinous layer over the whole liver: peritonitis. Can be caused by virulent *P. multocida*.
• Distomiasis: rare, only in 'backyard' rabbits fed with greens.

Spleen:
• About 4 cm long in a medium-sized rabbit.
• Significant enlargement (up to ten times normal weight): acute toxoplasmosis and salmonellosis; can be seen with rodentiosis and pasteurellosis also, though not very characteristic.
• Necrotic spots: indicate the same diseases; common with rodentiosis.

Urinary system:
• Precipitate in the bladder is normal (amorphous calcium carbonate crystals).
• Red colour of the urine is sometimes observed in rabbits. It is probably caused by a plant pigment and does not affect the health of the animal.
• Urolithiasis: rare.
• Inflammation of the bladder: hyperaemic bladder wall.
• Kidneys:
1 Infarcts = staphylococcosis (strains of human origin).
2 Uneven surface, pale patches: nosemosis (= encephalitozoonosis).
3 Scars on the surface: nosemosis.
• Inflammation: *P. multocida* can be the cause.

Female genital tract:
• Metritis: always examine the contents of the uterus. There are numerous possible causes.

Male genital tract:
- Purulent orchitis or epididymitis: *Pasteurella multocida.*

Spinal column:
- Examine lumbar vertebrae for trauma in connection with paralysis of hind limbs and incontinence.

12 / Microscopic and bacteriological examination as a diagnostic aid

Direct examination

Intestinal samples:
• Oöcysts and nematode eggs can be detected in direct smears. The smear is taken from places with visible lesions, or otherwise from the ileum, caecum and colon.
• No aetiological significance should be attached to the presence of more or less numerous *Saccharomyces* yeasts (cigar-shaped, or resembling a closed test tube with two or three flat little beads).
• Flagellates can sometimes be observed in the small intestine when the body is still warm. Their significance is unknown.

Liver abscesses:
• Direct smears show presence or absence of oöcysts of *Eimeria stiedae*.

Drops of bile:
• Examine as for liver abscesses.

May–Grünwald–Giemsa stainings

Heart blood samples and samples from the respiratory system:
• The interpretation is unreliable without additional bacteriological investigation. The presence of bipolar germs is not always an indication for the presence of *Pasteurella multocida,* as *Enterobacteriaceae* that have swarmed out of the intestinal system can also appear as bipolar rods after May–Grünwald–Giemsa staining. Conversely, often no bacteria can be seen in cases of septicaemia with *P. multocida.*

Scrapings from the ileal wall:
• Useful in checking for intracellular bacilli that stain irregularly and are an indication of Tyzzer's disease. This examination is only possible with animals that have just died. The following method has been recommended: smear preparations are air dried, fixed in methanol and then stained for 15 minutes with a 20% Giemsa solution in distilled water.

Impression smears of spleen and liver:
• Banana-shaped tachyzoids of *Toxoplasma gondii* can only be observed shortly after death (Plate 2). A positive result is very reliable, a negative one is not.
• A thin smear of liver homogenate can be stained quickly for the demonstration of *Bacillus piliformis* (Tyzzer's disease): first it is fixed for 30–60 seconds in methanol, and then stained in a 20% Giemsa solution in distilled water.

Carbolfuchsine staining of intestinal contents:
• Useful for the demonstration of *Cryptosporidium*. A small quantity of intestinal contents is mixed with an equal amount of a Ziehl–Neelsen carbolfuchsine solution, and smeared on a glass slide, so that a thin layer is formed. Immediately after drying, the preparation is covered with a drop of immersion oil and examined with a light microscope. The cryptosporidia appear as relatively large, light-breaking spherical organisms, lying in a coloured field. When the preparation has dried up completely they are more difficult to observe because they only appear as non-coloured spheres; the light-breaking effect is not seen any more.

Gram stainings

• Only with freshly dead animals.
• Ileum: massive and homogenous presence of short Gram-negative rods is an indication of *E. coli* infection; this occurs also clearly with neonatal coli-diarrhoea.
• Caecum: short Gram-negative rods do not always indicate an *E. coli* infection. The multiplication of *E. coli* can be secondary. Very curled Gram-positive rods indicate enterotoxaemia with *Clostridium spiroforme*.

Histological examination

This examination is indispensable in the diagnosis of *E. coli* intestinal infection, Tyzzer's disease, encephalitozoonosis and toxoplasmosis. Cryptosporidiosis and coccidiosis give also clearly recognizable histological lesions. In particular, material taken from the digestive and the central nervous systems must be fresh and must be fixed immediately after death. In practice this means that a sick animal must be humanely destroyed.

Bacteriological examination

Also here the material must be fresh. Freezing is an alternative when the material cannot be either immediately used or kept alive. The time elapsed between thawing and culturing must be kept to a minimum.

Practical applications: Differential diagnosis of respiratory infections and differential diagnosis of intestinal infections. In the first case, lung, heart and trachea must be preserved; in the second, the caecal contents must be kept.

13 / Diseases of the skin

Skin diseases caused by bacteria or fungi

Subcutaneous abscesses

Aetiology. Subcutaneous abscesses are almost always caused by *Pasteurella multocida* or *Staphylococcus aureus*. Usually *S. aureus* strains of human origin are involved although some farms are contaminated with strains of a special rabbit-pathogenic *S. aureus* type, in which case abscesses are frequently found in rabbits of all ages (see section on cutaneous staphylococcosis, below).

Symptoms. Painful local swelling. The abscesses can grow as large as hen's eggs. It is very difficult to obtain material from these abscesses by puncturing because rabbits form a very thick, toothpaste-like pus (Plate 3).

Treatment. Open widely, press the pus out, and rinse with an antiseptic or antibiotic solution. The latter is necessary for abscesses in the head region because antiseptics are too irritating for the nerves and blood vessels which are concentrated in this area. General treatment is seldom necessary.

Mastitis

Abscesses in the mammary glands are almost always caused by *Pasteurella multocida* or by *Staphylococcus aureus*.

A special form of mastitis which affects the skin on and around the teats is caused by rabbit-pathogenic *S. aureus* strains (see section on cutaneous staphylococcosis, below).

Cutaneous staphylococcosis

Occurrence. The disease is said to have spread extensively among the larger farms, principally in France, Italy and Hungary. It has also been reported in Belgium, England and Ireland.

Cause. Certain strains of *Staphylococcus aureus* of a biotype that is especially pathogenic for rabbits. These biotypes can only be identified in specialized laboratories.

Symptoms and course of the disease. In contrast to the disease which is caused by strains of human origin, it is not here a matter of sporadic cases, but of a form of the disease that is generally spread, especially in the breeding sections, among both the does and the young. Many of the does develop mastitis. The inflammation can be localized in the deeper-lying tissues of the udder, though a typical form is a purulent inflammation of the skin of the teats and the crown of the teats (Plate 4). Ulcerative pododermatitis (sore hocks) is frequently found both in does and in bucks (Plates 5 and 6). Such lesions can also be caused by other factors (see p. 48, Sore hocks) but in flocks contaminated with the rabbit-pathogenic staphylococci they are much more severe and frequent, and occur also in relatively young animals. Does with mastitis or sore hocks must be eliminated since they are no longer productive. Dissemination of the staphylococci from the superficial lesions also causes abdominal abscesses, pneumonia, septicaemia and many deaths.

Among the suckling young there is an abnormally high death rate caused both by agalactia in the mothers and by disease in the young themselves. The increased replacement percentage of the does, and especially the very high death rate (over 50%) among the baby rabbits, make it impossible for the rabbitries to operate at a profit.

Autopsy results

1 Among the very young rabbits (up to 10 days): widely spread skin inflammation of the type 'exudative dermatitis'. Superficial white foci the size of a pin-head are found on the wet skin (Plate 7).

2 Among those a little older (2–4 weeks): numerous pea-sized subcutaneous abscesses and purulent conjunctivitis; the eyes stick shut (Plate 8). Due to internal dissemination, abscesses will occasionally be found in the liver. Pneumonia is a very common sequella.

Diagnosis. Isolation of a *S. aureus* strain is not sufficient. Specialized laboratories can determine whether or not it is a rabbit strain.

Prognosis. Unfavourable for the rabbitry. The pathogenic *S. aureus* strains cannot be eliminated by treatment and disinfection, because they survive in the nares of infected rabbits.

Treatment. During treatment with antibiotics (for example, tetracycline 500 ppm in the feed) the problems disappear completely, but the disease breaks out again as soon as the treatment is stopped. The recommended solution is elimination of all animals, thorough disinfection and restarting with new breeding stock from a healthy farm.

Pseudomonas skin infection

Cause. Pseudomonas aeruginosa. This infection is actually a special form of 'moist dermatitis': dermatitis occasioned by the skin being kept wet or moist.

Occurrence. Mostly on rabbitries with automatic drinking water systems constructed with plastic pipes. Often these are very clean rabbitries that regularly use disinfectants.

Pathogenesis. The infection occurs on skin areas that are continuously wet, for example: under the dewlap, or on the back when the animal always lies under the drinking nipple.

Symptoms and lesions. Moist skin, loss of hair, inflammation of skin. Sometimes the hair around the affected zone has a greenish-blue colour. The underlying muscle tissue can also have a green colour (Plate 9).

Diagnosis. Isolation of *Pseudomonas aeruginosa.*

Treatment

1 Operational: letting the drinking water line dry out well. Disinfection of these lines with chlorine is good, but the disinfectant must be concentrated enough (chloramine 0.5%).

2 Individual: topical application of preparations containing gentamicin. Gentamicin can also be administered systemically (only by injection).

Treponematosis (syphilis, spirochaetosis; see Chapter 17)

With spirochaetosis, dermatitis of the nose is also found, in addition to the cutaneous lesions on the genitals. There is also loss of hair, and in chronic cases the skin appears dry and scaly. There may also be scabs. Spirochaetosis is extremely rare.

Dermatomycosis

Cause. Microsporum canis as well as *Trichophyton mentagrophytes* have been reported to cause epidemics in rabbitries.

Symptoms and signs. The lesions appear mostly on the head, ears and paws. There is complete or partial alopecia and the skin appears dry and scaly; slight itching is typical (Plate 10). The lesions may be secondarily invaded by *Streptococcus pneumoniae* of human origin, and this causes more severe and purulent infections.

Diagnosis. Isolation of the fungus from the skin scrapings and hair collected around the edge of the lesions. *Microsporum canis* isolated from rabbits forms a yellow to orange pigment in cultures.

Treatment

1 Hygiene: regular burning with a gas-burner of wool and hair left hanging in the cages.

2 Adding griseofulvin to the feed is recommended only in exceptional cases since it is so expensive. The best dosage is 0.750 g per kg feed for 14 days. A clinical cure can be accomplished by spraying in the sheds with an enilconazole solution (50 mg/m floor area, twice a week for 20 weeks). Particularly, the walls and ceiling should be thoroughly sprayed. Such expensive methods of treatment are financially justifiable only for valuable breeding animals.

Skin diseases caused by parasites

Ear mange (synonym: ear canker)

Ear canker is one of the most common infections with 'backyard' rabbits. The parasite is also often found in pets. On industrial rabbit farms it is less important.

Cause. Psoroptes cuniculi.

Symptoms. Itching ears; the animals shake their heads and scratch. An otoscope is usually not needed to see the lesions: greyish-white crusts in the ear canals and the earlobe. Sometimes the skin in the vicinity of the ear is also affected.

Diagnosis. Typical macroscopic lesions and/or microscopic examination of the crusts for the mite or its eggs.

Differential diagnosis. Sarcoptes scabiei also causes mange on the head, but spreads further over the whole body. *Sarcoptes scabiei* is not commonly found in rabbits.

Treatment

1 Topical: A mixture of mineral oil with an acaricide is sufficient. With severely affected animals, the crusts have to be removed with a mild detergent solution before local treatment is started. Commercially available antibiotic-acaricide preparations used to treat ear mange in cats and dogs are also good. Local treatments must be applied several times.

2 Injections: Ivermectin can be applied: 400 µg/kg body weight, via the subcutaneous route. This treatment must be repeated once, 6 days later. Administering ivermectin is simpler than local treatment,

especially with serious cases where the animals are suffering a great deal and resist handling, and also when large numbers have to be treated.

Fur mites (very common)

Two types occur: *Cheyletiella parasitovorax* and *Listrophorus gibbus*. Both are often considered apathogenic, but this appears not always to be the case.

On white rabbits they can be seen with the naked eye when present in great numbers; they appear as small black dots, especially on the back of the rabbit. The damage they do is in fact quite modest: loss of hair on the back, scaly skin, itching. This is especially a problem for raisers of show rabbits. Affected animals may also show signs of restlessness. Many other animals do not seem to be bothered by the parasites.

Treatment. Dichlorvos strips in the sheds. If necessary, the animals can also be treated topically with an insecticide.

Other mites

Dermanyssus gallinae (red fowl mite) may also attack mammals. This parasite can cause severe restlessness in rabbits that are housed together with fowl, especially in poorly constructed, unhygienic sheds.

Lice and fleas

Lice and fleas do not occur commonly with domesticated rabbits. The European rabbit flea, *Spilopsyllus cuniculi*, however, is found frequently among wild rabbits and is an important vector for myxomatosis. Domestic rabbits that run loose and dig tunnels can catch this flea if they come into contact with wild rabbits. It can be found in and around the auricles.

Occasionally, pet rabbits are infected with cat fleas.

Viral skin diseases

Myxomatosis

Cause. The myxoma virus belongs to the group called pox viruses. This virus is endemic in a native South American rabbit species, in which it causes a mild disease. When it infected imported European rabbits, however, the result was nearly 100% mortality. In the 1950s the virus was intentionally introduced in Australia where the European rabbit had previously, and just as artificially, been introduced and had created a plague by itself. By accident, the virus also came to Europe and in the course of a few years had spread over the whole continent and Great Britain, decimating the wild rabbit population.

Epidemiology. The disease occurs with both wild and domesticated rabbits and with European hares, although the hares are quite resistant to it.

Transmission is possible via direct or indirect contact, or via vectors. It is mechanical in nature, so that every rabbit parasite is a potential vector. Mosquitoes and rabbit fleas are particularly important in this respect. On the European continent the mosquito is the principle vector, which explains the obvious seasonality in the frequency of myxomatosis.

Symptoms. The original form of the virus was extremely virulent and produced an acute illness with 100% mortality. The lesions are typical: oedema of the head, eyelids and genitals. The appetite usually remains normal until shortly before death. Purulent blepharo-conjunctivitis, with swelling of the eyelids, is a constant symptom and leads to the typical blindness (Plate 11).

With the chronic or nodular form, which is now common, oedematous swellings called pseudo-tumours develop after several days, especially on the ears, nose and paws (Plate 12). This form can heal spontaneously: the pseudo-tumours regress, leaving scabs which later disappear.

In France another disease has been diagnosed which is also caused by a variant of the myxoma virus but which only produces respiratory difficulties and pneumonia. Snuffles typically develop, usually complicated with pasteurellae, which are present on every rabbitry. This disease is not communicated via vectors, but through direct contact. In other countries the respiratory form has not yet been noted, though in some cases the differential diagnosis with pasteurellosis can be difficult.

Diagnosis. The symptoms are so typical in the acute and the nodular form that further investigations are not necessary.

Differential diagnosis of the chronic and respiratory forms
1 With treponematosis: the regressed pseudo-tumours of the atten-

uated form of myxomatosis can resemble the lesions of treponematosis. Treponematosis is much rarer, and when it does occur it is much more chronic.

2 With snuffles: whenever many animals on a farm suddenly show symptoms of snuffles, combined with conjunctivitis, the peri-anal zone of the affected animals should be checked for swelling (the last symptom is typical for myxomatosis). This should be checked even when *Pasteurellae* are isolated from the nasal cavity, because many animals are healthy carriers of this germ.

Treatment. To treat infected rabbitries, it is advised to humanely destroy the diseased animals and to remove them in such a way as to form no source of infection for the others. They are unfit for consumption, although the virus itself is not pathogenic for human beings.

Symptomatic treatment can be tried with pet or hobby rabbits. Treating rabbits suffering from the acute form is, however, discouraging: they survive for 2 weeks and continue eating and drinking, but eventually die with severe breathing difficulties. They should be humanely destroyed whenever possible. Rabbits with the nodular form may survive. Palliative treatment (for example, eyedrops, antibiotic injections) can be provided.

The most economical course of action in a unit which breeds rabbits for meat, then, is immediately to slaughter those animals that have attained enough weight, and to vaccinate the young and the breeding stock (see below: Prevention). Contrary to commonly accepted opinion, such a vaccination procedure on an already infected rabbitry produces good results. Care must be taken to change the needle after each hutch or nest since otherwise the procedure may actually spread the disease. Myxomatosis has an incubation period of 7–14 days. Immunity is fully built up 8 days after vaccination. Thus the raiser should be aware that up to 2 weeks after vaccination new animals can still develop the disease.

Disinfection. The virus is very resistant to dryness and cold, but not to heat and light. Good disinfectants include formalin, hypochlorite and sodium hydroxide (8%). The virus can survive for several months in vectors (fleas in the case of wild rabbits), but also in overwintering mosquitoes.

Prevention. The most economical means of prevention is usually to control the vectors by applying insecticides for mosquitoes and preventing direct or indirect contact with wild rabbits. For small-scale raisers this is often not possible. Also on some farms with deep-well manure removal systems it is impossible to combat the vectors efficiently.

In such cases, vaccination is recommended, although the cost is rather high. Until recently, the vaccines that were most commonly used consisted of living fibroma virus which induced cross-immunity with the myxoma virus; sometimes it was combined with an adjuvant. Immunity induced with this type of vaccines, however, lasted only a few months. Breeding animals housed in threatened sheds should be inoculated twice a year: the best months are February to March and July to August. Pregnant does, or does with newborn young, are best not vaccinated, unless the contamination risk is very high (that is in infected rabbitries).

During the last few years, different live homologous vaccines have been developed. The first one was developed in France; the attenuated strain SG 33, however, had an immunodepressive action, so it was not safe in the field because of the high rate of animals in which subclinical pasteurella infections became clinical. For this reason it is no longer available.

A second homologous vaccine has been developed in Hungary; the virus strain is MM-16005. It is now in common use but it must be injected intramuscularly and not subcutaneously, which causes severe swelling. The protection lasts for at least a year. In young animals, however, it is less active, and in the unweaned (less than 5 weeks old) it can produce a serious reaction. It is advised to vaccinate only rabbits older than 5 weeks unless in a contaminated environment where immediate protection is required. The vaccine has a high safety level and does not affect production rates of breeding females, nor the incidence of pneumonia in farms infected by pasteurella.

A third vaccine has been produced in Spain and consists of the homologous strain Léon-162. It was tested thoroughly in the laboratory and in the field: it is very safe and procures a long-lasting immunity. It is often asked for by hunters because it is said to spread from animal to animal; in this case it could be able to protect a population of wild rabbits. It was indeed demonstrated that non-vaccinated rabbits showed sero-conversion against the vaccine strain when they had been in close contact with recently vaccinated ones; it was not examined whether they were protected against infection, though this was probably the case. It is doubtful whether the same event will take place on a large scale in natural conditions.

Still another homologous vaccine has been developed in Italy. So far few data are available on this.

It can be concluded that vaccines consisting of homologous attenuated strains are more active than vaccines prepared from Shope's fibroma virus. Since comparative investigations have not been carried out, a 'best choice' cannot be indicated. All homologous vaccines that are now available in Europe can be considered active and safe when the instructions for use are followed.

Fibromatosis

Fibromatosis is a benign disease of *Sylvilagus floridanus*, an American rabbit species. Under normal circumstances fibromatosis does not occur with European rabbits. The virus, which is called Shope's virus, is important, however, because it is the principal component of the heterologous vaccines for myxomatosis. Some strains produce an extremely widespread illness among the newborn, so it is recommended not to vaccinate rabbits with the fibroma virus before 3 weeks of age.

Predominant traumatic skin diseases

Sore hocks (ulcerative pododermatitis)

See Plates 5 and 6.

Cause. Complex. Various factors play a role: body weight of the animal, thickness of the skin, thickness of the fur on the foot soles, quality of the wire mesh or litter on the floor. Most rabbit breeds are not suited for wire mesh floors. Selected strains and breeds intended for meat production should have wire mesh floors, since it is not economical to keep them on straw. Rabbits with a very delicate skin can develop sore hocks even when kept on straw, especially when they are old and heavy.

The earliest traumatic lesions are very small and sometimes not even visible, but they almost always become infected with staphylococci. In rabbitries infected with the special rabbit pathogenic *Staphylococcus aureus* strains there will be an abnormally high incidence of sore hocks, even among the younger animals (see section on cutaneous staphylococcosis, above).

Symptoms and lesions. Ulcers on the footpad(s). Abscesses and lymphangitis can develop. The animals become restless; their appetite falls off; they lose weight and stop breeding. The staphylococci can disseminate into the abdominal organs; human strains often cause typical renal infarcts. Commercial animals are usually slaughtered before they become totally worthless or die from generalized staphylococcosis.

Prevention. The bedding of rabbits that are housed on straw must be kept dry and changed regularly.

Only breeds and crossbreeds that are suited for it can be kept on wire mesh; otherwise there will always be problems with older animals. Some breeders use plastic grilles, which can be cleaned and disinfected easily, for the adult does and bucks. Only highly finished wire mesh that is designed for rabbits should be used.

Treatment. Recommended only for valuable breeding stock and for pet and show rabbits. The wounds should be treated carefully with disinfecting ointments. Soft and dry bedding should be provided during healing.

Prognosis Poor; treatment must be continued until complete recovery, and relapses are frequent.

Self-plucking of wool (hairballs, gastric trichobezoars, wool block)

This behaviour is physiologically triggered, in the case of does, shortly before partus. They pluck their own fur, mainly from the breast and around the milk glands, and use it to line their nest. When the animals groom themselves it is also normal for them to swallow some hair. This hair is expelled with the dung, making the droppings stick together, and can most easily be observed during the moulting period. Older animals of either sex that are kept in wire cages, however, often begin to lick and clean themselves excessively. The hair they swallow clumps together in the stomach where it interferes with digestion and can even clog the passage out of the stomach. Whenever this type of doe is mated it usually dies before the end of gestation. Other animals start wasting away or may die suddenly of some complication such as an obstruction of the small intestine or a tear in the stomach. This phenomenon occurs more frequently during the moulting season and is especially common with long-haired breeds. In Angora farms it is one of the most significant causes of financial loss.

Post-mortem findings. Presence of hair mixed with food in the stomach. Fatty degeneration of the liver.

Diagnosis. Palpation. Contrast radiography (only for pets or valuable animals).

Prognosis. Poor for the individual animal.

Treatment. Twenty millilitres of paraffin oil orally twice a day for at least 1 week. After administering the oil, gentle massage of the stomach for 3 minutes helps to break up the hairball.

Risks:

1 Obstruction of the small intestine.

2 Tearing of the liver.

Others suggest that the administration of 10 ml of raw pineapple juice, two or three times per day, will help. Pineapple contains an enzyme, bromelin, which breaks down the hairball. Direct administration of such enzymes (bromelin or papain) is perhaps even more effective. Simultaneously, hay should be provided, to promote the passage of the hairs through the intestines.

Prevention. Supply hay or straw. Relieve boredom. Changing the diurnal light rhythm may help.

Fur chewing of cage mates

Occurrence. Young broiler rabbits in batteries.

Cause. Deviant behaviour on the part of one or more rabbits in the affected cage. They attack another rabbit which crouches with its head lowered, while each attacker plucks out a few tufts of fur, which it eats up completely. This deviant behaviour seems to grow out of boredom and irritation though other factors, such as light intensity, also play a role.

Lesions and symptoms. Bald spots on forehead, neck and back. The phenomenon occurs only in one or a few cages. The number of rabbits affected may vary from one to several per cage. Usually at least one rabbit is unaffected: this one is the offender.

Treatment. Provide hay and straw and reduce light intensity. Remove the offender.

Malignant tumours

Mammary gland carcinoma

'Cystic disease' refers to a mammary gland carcinoma, which is rarely found in older females, and which is characterized by the presence of multiple cysts in the mammary tissue.

14 / Diseases of the eye

Chronic conjunctivitis

Cause. This type of conjunctivitis is usually ascribed to *Pasteurella multocida. P. multocida* is, however, not always isolated; other causes probably exist also.

Symptoms. The exudate is serous to mucopurulent. The eyelids are swollen and the conjunctiva is red. Continuous flow of exudate can cause a partial or total loss of hair downwards from the medial corner of the eye (Plate 13).

Treatment. Antibiotic eyesalve or drops. Check the ventilation in the shed; eliminate draughts, excessive ammonia concentrations and other irritations. After treatment the symptoms can return because of the continuous presence of the causative agent in the nasal cavity.

Myxomatosis

Myxomatosis produces a purulent blepharoconjunctivitis. In the nodular form the myxomatous tumours also typically develop on the eyelids (see Chapter 13).

Hereditary glaucoma ('Buphthalmia' or 'ox eye')

Cause. A recessive genetic factor which occurs often in New Zealand Whites (Plate 14). This factor causes a decrease in the outflow of aqueous from the anterior eye chamber. It is probable that the initial cause is a deficient vitamin A metabolism.

Symptoms and lesions. These can appear as early as 2 or 3 weeks after birth, though usually not until later. Nevertheless most infected rabbits develop the symptoms at a relatively early age (3–5 months old).

In the early stage the anterior eye chamber is enlarged, and the cornea is flattened, but still fairly clear. Later it gradually becomes opaque. This may be followed by ulceration and rupture of the cornea. The eyeball may be enlarged when the disease occurs at an early age.

Prognosis and treatment. The condition cannot be treated, but pet

51

rabbits can survive even when both eyes are affected. The same holds true for broiler rabbits, which can be brought to slaughter weight without problems. Raisers of show rabbits, however, should be warned that the condition is hereditary.

Eyelid abnormalities of unknown aetiology

In some colonies a distinct eyelid abnormality may occur in several nests. It is not clear whether this aberration is hereditary or is a sequel of an infection at a very early age. The edge of the upper eyelid, where the eyelashes grow, is not straight but rather crenated. This produces the same effect as entropion: purulent keratitis and conjunctivitis as a result of irritation by the eyelashes. The abnormality is either uni- or bilateral and occurs in several animals in each affected nest. An abnormality of the eyelashes that produces similar effects has been observed in the Rex breeds.

The symptoms become noticeable only at the age of 2 weeks when the eyes open. From then on it becomes progressively worse, although very mild cases can heal spontaneously.

Treatment. A surgical procedure like that for entropion in dogs can effect improvement or even complete healing. Such costly surgery is indicated only for pet rabbits.

In broiler rabbits, antibiotic eyesalves bring enough improvement to enable many of the animals to grow to slaughter weight without problems.

15 / Diseases of the respiratory system

Snuffles (coryza, rhinitis, sinusitis) and complications of chronic pasteurellosis (purulent pleuropneumonia, otitis media, abscesses, peritonitis, metritis, mastitis). Enzootic pneumonia

Occurrence. In practically all large-scale rabbitries, and most of the smaller ones. Pasteurellosis is also a problem in most laboratory rabbit units and in Angora rabbit farms.

Cause. Pasteurella multocida strains of low to moderate virulence; highly virulent strains cause acute pasteurellosis (see Chapter 19). Also, though rarely, *Pseudomonas aeruginosa* may be involved.

Most *Pasteurella multocida* strains from rabbits require a bacteriological medium that contains serum or blood for growth. There is no good selective medium for the rabbit strains of *P. multocida* and thus it is not easily isolated from contaminated material (for example, out of the nasal cavity). Isolation from cadavers only works when they are either relatively fresh or have been frozen immediately after death.

There are two capsule types among *P. multocida* strains from rabbits: A-type strains form colonies of various sizes which require rich media for growth, while D-type strains produce colonies of uniform size and are less exacting in their growth requirement. D-types are generally more virulent. This virulence cannot be determined from the bacteriological characteristics, but it can be measured using the LD 50 determination in mice. The virulence for rabbits and mice runs parallel.

Most *P. multocida* strains from rabbits belong to serogroups 3 or 11 or 12 (Heddleston's somatic antigens). They share also common antigenic determinants. *P. multocida* also causes disease in other animal species (poultry, swine and cattle) or belongs to the nasal flora without causing troubles (cats) but these strains are different from those which cause snuffles and enzootic pneumonia in rabbits. Nevertheless there are exceptional strains which are extremely virulent for different animal species, such as serotype 1 strains which are pathogenic for mice, rabbits and poultry. Such strains can occasionally be isolated from rabbits which have died of septicaemia but are entirely different from the 'typical rabbit *P. multocida*' strains.

Symptoms. Typical snuffles does not occur in very young animals

53

in which the sinuses have not yet developed. Nevertheless, un-weaned young can show pneumonia caused by *P. multocida*, though this is not frequent. Snuffles is more of a problem in breeding stock than in broilers and is seen more in closed sheds than in hutches in the open air.

The most characteristic symptom is mucopurulent nasal discharge; affected rabbits sneeze and cough. The external nares are soiled with dried exudate. Since rabbits frequently clean themselves, the latter symptom is not always evident, but in that case the hairs of the inner edge of the forepaws are wet and stick together. Rabbits can have chronic snuffles without apparently suffering much from it. The possible complications include pneumonia, otitis media and interna (which can cause torticollis), pericarditis, metritis and subcutaneous abscesses. The morbidity and mortality depend on, among other things, the virulence of the *Pasteurella* strain involved and climatological conditions.

Lesions. Presence of pus in the nasal cavities and sinuses. When complicated: purulent tracheitis, purulent pleuropneumonia, purulent pericarditis, tracheitis, subcutaneous abscesses, metritis, mastitis and other localizations of purulent conditions (Plates 15 and 16).

Treatment. Individual treatment of rabbits infected with snuffles is not very effective. All *Pasteurella* strains from rabbits are sensitive *in vitro* to the usual antibiotics. Even the highest doses of these antibiotics, however, have no effect on the bacterial populations in the nasal cavities, although they may prevent possible complications during the period of treatment.

Mass treatment of large farms should include:

1 Elimination of diseased animals. They spread the illness through sneezing, are less productive, and infect their young at a very early age. Eliminating all *Pasteurella* carriers is an impossible task, though, because many are asymptomatic and because bacteriological examination of nasal swabs often gives false negative results. In addition, *Pasteurella*-free breeding stock is extremely difficult to find. Recently, an ELISA test has been developed which should be more effective to detect *P. multocida* carriers.

2 Controlling the climate: minimal temperature fluctuations, correct humidity levels, good ventilation and no draughts. It is a well established fact that extreme fluctuations of temperature can trigger latent infections. As explained in Chapter 6, Housing and hygiene, rabbits can withstand cold very well. The ideal temperature in a

rabbit shed is 16°C; with lower temperatures feed consumption rises, though adult animals suffer no ill effects. Every stress situation, however, such as humid bedding or high temperature fluctuations, and also shearing of Angoras and even intensive breeding with does in large-scale farms increases the risk of pasteurellosis. Ventilation is also important. Experimental studies have shown that the infection takes hold more easily and produces a more serious illness when the ammonia concentration is high, which is common in closed sheds.

Vaccination. *Pasteurella multocida* strains from rabbits belong to two capsule types, several somatic serotypes and several biotypes, but the great majority carry the somatic antigens 3 and 12, and capsule type A is more frequent than capsule type D. This is important because cross-immunity is higher between strains belonging to the same serotype. Nevertheless test vaccines are more effective against infection with homologous than with heterologous strains, even when these have the same serotype. This was proven through the measurement of protection in experimental tests with mice.

Effectiveness in counteracting the snuffles or chronic form of pasteurellosis has never been established because the snuffles disease is difficult to reproduce. Also vaccination trials in the field, in farms snuffering from pasteurellosis, have not convincingly proved the advantages of vaccination against snuffles. On the other hand, homologous killed vaccines are quite effective against the acute form of pasteurellosis (see Chapter 19, Systemic diseases). Vaccinated rabbits are protected for at least 6 months. The addition of adjuvants to the inactivated bacterial suspension is not necessary to obtain good protection.

Local vaccination reactions (foreign-body granulomas) can develop. These seldom grow very large and break open. Usually the granulomas remain small and are cut away with the skin at slaughter time. It is only with show rabbits that they may be a problem.

Live, streptomycin-dependent or temperature-dependent *P. multocida* strains may be more effective vaccines against snuffles, but have up till now not been commercialized.

Bordetella bronchiseptica infection

Practically all rabbits are infected with *B. bronchiseptica*. They usually experience very few ill effects from it, although histological lesions are present in the trachea and bronchi. Pneumonia caused by

B. bronchiseptica is very rare. The infection can by no means be considered of great economical importance.

Bordetella bronchiseptica is probably the cause of 'snoring' rabbits. These are rabbits with loud breathing but without a runny nose. Even this condition seems to create no problem for the animals. It disappears when treated with tetracycline. Presumably it can also disappear spontaneously.

Staphylococcus aureus infection

Generalized staphylococcosis, which is usually caused by special strains pathogenic for rabbits, often expresses itself in the form of pneumonia, both in young as well as in adult animals. To differentiate it from pneumonia caused by *Pasteurella multocida*, a bacteriological examination is required. Pneumonia caused by *P. multocida* is usually a purulent pleuropneumonia, while that caused by *S. aureus* is most often characterized by numerous small abscesses in the lungs.

Pseudomonas infection

Infection with *Pseudomonas aeruginosa* can also lead to coryza, pneumonia and death. Symptoms can resemble snuffles very closely. Sporadic cases usually occur in installations, large and small, which employ watering systems fitted with plastic pipes. The disease is seen more often in laboratory rabbits than in rabbits of other origins.

Treatment. See section on *Pseudomonas* skin infection in Chapter 13.

'Foreign-body pneumonia'

In about 60% of the cases of caecal impaction–mucoid enteropathy complex (see Chapter 16) a special lung inflammation is found that is not caused by the known pathogenic bacteria. This pneumonia is limited to the apical lobes of the lung. It does not have a purulent character. The affected portion of the lung is red and it sinks in water; the border with the healthy lung tissue is sharply delineated. There is spumous fluid in the trachea. Shortly before death, fluid, possibly stomach contents, runs out the mouth and nose, which is often mistakenly taken as a sign of snuffles. Histological examination reveals that plant cells are present in the trachea, the large bronchial tubes and the lung tissue. Thus the name, 'foreign-body pneumonia' has been used for this condition. The true origin of this form of pneumonia is, however, still unknown, as is the aetiology and pathogenesis of the whole complex.

Myxomatosis

Rabbits suffering from the acute forms of myxomatosis sniff and show signs of dyspnoea. Moreover, on a few large French rabbitries a pneumonia has been discovered which is caused by a mutant myxomatosis virus possessing only very limited dermatotropic characteristics. This disease is described in the section on myxomatosis in Chapter 13.

16 / Diseases of the digestive system

Introduction

'Enteritis complex', 'non-specific enteritis', dysentery', 'mucoid enteritis' . . . these are all names for diseases which involve the whole digestive system and for which, for a long time, aetiologies were quite unknown. As such, they constituted the greatest hindrance to the development of rabbit raising for meat on an industrial scale.

On small rabbitries and in small colonies the principal causes of death are coccidiosis and a few general diseases, including acute pasteurellosis, pseudotuberculosis, salmonellosis and myxomatosis. On industrial rabbitries, by contrast, hygienic conditions are better (a) because of the wire mesh floors, (b) because rodents and insects for the most part are under control, and (c) because hay and greens are excluded from the diet.

In the industrial situation, on the other hand, there is (a) heightened stress due to the intensive or semi-intensive breeding rhythm, (b) a higher population density, and (c) the use of high-energy feeds which produce not only faster growth, but also in some circumstances a rise in the percentage of intestinal disorders. Moreover, there is the necessity of regularly purchasing new breeding stock, which brings with it the possibility of new infectious agents to which the present population has no resistance. This danger is especially high in operations which use hybrid rabbits. In the opinion of the author, the knowledge of the aetiology and prevention of rabbit diseases is not yet advanced enough to justify the use of this expensive breeding method. The profit to be gained through the higher number of young per doe and the more rapid growth is usually offset by the high losses that all rabbitries are subject to. In addition to these expected losses, farms using hybrids will have a heightened risk of imported infections.

In recent years much research has been done in this field. Because of the advances that have been made, many of the cases that previously were classified as 'non-specific enteritis' can now be diagnosed aetiologically. An aetiological diagnosis is in many cases only possible when an animal showing the typical symptoms is brought live to the diagnostic laboratory. Some aetiologies can only be demonstrated through histological examination of intestines that have been fixed in formalin immediately after death. When a live animal cannot be taken to the laboratory, the veterinarian can perform an autopsy on location at the rabbitry itself and fix 2–3 cm long pieces of duodenum, ileum and colon in a 10% solution of formaldehyde within 15 minutes of death. A sample of the caecum contents should also be taken for bacteriological and parasitological examination; the part intended for bacteriological examination should be kept in the deep freeze in order to prevent the proliferation of saprophytic germs. The anamnesis and the necropsy report are indispensable aids in establishing a good diagnosis.

Essential data that must be included in the anamnesis are:
• Age of the infected animals.
• Morbidity and mortality.
• Hyperacute, acute or chronic course of the disease.
• The occurrence of stunted animals or frequent weight losses.

The autopsy report must at minimum contain:
• General condition of the body (well fed, cachectic . . .)
• Type and location of inflammatory lesions in the intestines.
• Consistency of the intestinal contents.
• Appearance of lungs, spleen, liver, kidneys.

Digestive-tract disorders of bacterial origin

Escherichia coli infections

General

In human medicine, *E. coli* that cause enteric infections and diarrhoea have been subdivided into three major groups: enterotoxigenic *E. coli* (ETEC); entero-invasive *E. coli* (EIEC); and enteropathogenic *E. coli* (EPEC). Besides these, the recently discovered enterohaemorrhagic *E. coli* (EHEC) are sometimes considered a fourth distinct group.

This subdivision is based mainly on the virulence mechanism of the causative *E. coli* strains involved. ETEC act by elaborating enterotoxins, which cause hypersecretion of water without seriously damaging the intestinal epithelium. EIEC invade the intestinal cells, just as their name suggests. The exact mechanism used by the 'classical' EPEC, which cause chronic diarrhoea in human infants, is not known. The cytotoxins which they produce and which, as opposed to enterotoxins, damage and destroy the intestinal epithelial cells, are probably responsible for the ill effects. They share this faculty with EHEC, of which the only known serotype causes food intoxication in adult human beings.

In veterinary medicine, only ETEC are well known. The most important infections caused by them include neonatal diarrhoea in calves and pigs.

On the other hand, all *E. coli* strains that cause diarrhoea in rabbits are comparable to the 'classical EPEC' of human medicine. Therefore, they are called 'EPEC-like', or simply 'rabbit EPEC'. The name 'attaching and effacing *E. coli*' (AEEC) is also an appropriate term. The last name refers to the typical histological lesions that are seen with rabbit and human EPEC infections: they attach to and efface the microvillous border of the intestinal epithelium.

Just like ETEC, EPEC need an adhesin as an additional virulence characteristic. K88, K99 and others are well known as adhesins of pig and calf ETEC. Adhesins of rabbit EPEC have not been studied much, with the exception of one type strain called RDEC-1 (see below).

Escherichia coli diarrhoea in newborn and unweaned rabbits

Occurrence. Neonatal diarrhoea in rabbits is not rare, but because of the low value of the individual animals veterinary help is not often asked for. The disease is encountered in large-scale farms as well as in small units.

Cause. In Belgium, where the first cases have been described, only *E. coli* serotype O109 has been isolated from cases of neonatal diarrhoea. In France other serotypes are mentioned but since no experimental infections have been performed with them, their significance remains uncertain. The isolated O109 strains do not form enterotoxins (in contrast to the calf and piglet neonatal strains) and they are not invasive, but they do attach themselves *in vivo* to the brush border of the intestinal wall cells. This attachment can also be demonstrated *in vitro* with fixed intestinal villi of newborn rabbits.

Symptoms. The disease is found in rabbits aged 1–14 days. They have a watery diarrhoea that discolours the belly and the posterior part of the body yellow. Usually the whole nest is infected at the same time and they all die. The disease often occurs in the form of an outbreak in which numerous nests are affected. Nests of does that have previously had an infected nest usually remain healthy.

Lesions. The first thing noticed at the necropsy is the stomach, which is overful with undigested milk. The intestinal contents are watery and thin. Very young rabbits are completely wet, while those that are a little older merely have a dirtied, yellow posterior. In newborns the infection develops as septicaemica and abscesses can also form in the liver.

Diagnosis. Isolation of *E. coli* in large quantities from the intestinal contents of rabbits less than 2 weeks of age is actually sufficient since this bacterium is not normally found at this age in the intestinal tract of rabbits. Histological examination can demonstrate the attachment of the coccobacilli. A freshly dead or killed animal is necessary for both bacteriological and histological examinations.

Differential diagnosis. Other causes of death in newborn rabbits include neglect, agalactia in the doe, staphylococcosis, hypothermia and nest watering by the doe; see Chapter 21.

Treatment. All the young of each nest must be individually dosed with oral antibiotics. Resistance to antibiotics is not rare with rabbit EPEC; an antibiogram is indicated. Treatment should continue until a few days after the disappearance of the symptoms. A rabbit which is a few days old weighs about 100 g. Oral suspensions for use in piglets or human infants can be administered to rabbit kits (see Chapter 22).

Escherichia coli diarrhoea in weaned rabbits

Occurrence. Probably the most frequent intestinal disease in large-scale rabbit farms all over the European continent.

Cause. Several *E. coli* serotypes of varying virulence exist which all cause diarrhoea in weaned rabbits. They belong to different 'biotypes' or serotypes. The serotype O15:H- (non-motile strains, 'biotype' 3) which has been isolated in the US, Holland and Belgium, is very virulent. In addition, there are O103, O109, O132 and perhaps other sertotypes which have been studied in France, Belgium and Hungary. Many of those strains contain the flagellar antigen H2; some contain H7. All these strains are non-invasive and form no enterotoxins, but they do attach to the brush border of the cells of the intestinal wall. Just like the neonatal strains, they belong to the EPEC group. Attachment *in vitro* has also been demonstrated for some of the weaned rabbit EPEC. In laboratory conditions, O15:H- strains are only pathogenic for weaned rabbits; in exceptional cases it is found in diarrrhoeal younger rabbits in the field.

Other strains are pathogenic for weaned and infant rabbits, as was shown by experimental infections. To this group belong a number of strains that possess the flagellar antigen H2, and all show identical biochemical characteristics.

Symptoms. Coli-enteritis causes moderate to high losses among weaned broiler rabbits. The appetite falls off sharply and the animals have a watery diarrhoea. Scattered individual animals die suddenly, usually as a result of intestinal invagination. Most of the infected animals, however, die only after several days of illness, usually completely wasted. Some rabbits recover but remain anywhere from slightly to far behind in growth compared to healthy animals of the same age. Rabbitries which are infected with the O15:H- serotype may experience mortality rates of 50% and higher. Most other serotypes are much less virulent and cause outbreaks with only occasionally high death rates.

Lesions. The lesions are limited to the caecum and large intestine, whose contents are watery, bad smelling and light brown to blood-tinged, but seldom haemorrhagic. The caecal wall may be slightly or severely inflamed. Longitudinal haemorrhages may be seen in the outer wall of the caecum; this is also called 'the paint-brush' type of bleeding (Plates 17 and 18). Intestinal invagination or rectal prolapse may be observed in animals that die suddenly.

Diagnosis. Observing attached *E. coli* by means of histological examination. For this, a freshly killed animal is required. Even though the caecum contents of healthy adult rabbits contain little or no *E. coli* ($<10^3$/g), the isolation of great numbers of *E. coli* here constitutes no proof. A secondary multiplication of apathogenic *E. coli* may occur in connection with all types of intestinal inflammation. High numbers of *E. coli* in the ileum of a rabbit that has died recently are a good indication of *E. coli* diarrhoea. A combination of semi-quantitative estimations in the caecum, ileum and jejunum by simply inoculating a loopful of contents on MacConkey agar provides still a more reliable method: confluent growth from all three sites is required. Serotyping of the isolated *E. coli* strains remains so far a tool for research only, not for diagnosis. Biotyping is a valuable aid, but must be interpreted in combination with the histological examination (see Table 16.1) and differential diagnosis.

Differential diagnosis. Coli-diarrhoea must be differentiated from enterotoxaemia, coccidiosis, Tyzzer's disease and mucoid enteropathy. Since most rabbit farms suffer from more than one intestinal

Table 16.1 Biochemical characteristics of rabbit EPEC strains, related to
serotype and pathogenicity for infant and weaned rabbits

	Biotype				
	1	2	3	4	8
Serotype(s)	0109:H2	0109:H2 0128:H2 0132:H2 0128:H−	015:H−	?	0103
Pathogenicity for weaner	Low	Moderate	High	High	High
Pathogenicity for unweaned	High	High	None	None	?
Motility	+	+ or −	−	+	+
Ornithine decarboxylase	+	+	+	+	+
Cellobiose	−	−	−	−	−
Dulcitol	−	Slowly+	+	−	+
Raffinose	+	+	+	+	+
Rhamnose	+	+	+	−	−
Sorbose	−	−	+	+	−
Sucrose	+	+	+	+	+

infection, it is advisable to examine several animals in order to
determine the most important cause of losses.

It is also important to detect which type of EPEC strain is the
cause of the problem. For this, it is necessary to type the strains
beyond the species level in biotypes and/or serotypes. Biochemical
characteristics, in relation to pathogenical properties and serotype,
are listed in Table 16.1.

Treatment. When a rabbitry is infected with the less virulent
biotype 2 strains, hygienic measures should be sufficient to limit the
mortality rate. At the time of outbreak, treatment with antibiotics is
indicated; tetracycline, neomycin, nitrofurantoin and polymyxins
can be tried, but neomycin is considered most effective. An
antibiogram is necessary because many strains are resistant to the
commonly used antibiotics in rabbits. The choice of antibiotics is
already restricted (see section on indirect toxicity of antibiotics,
Chapter 22). Hygienic measures should be taken to lower the
infection risk: separation of the rabbits into compartments which can

be regularly emptied and disinfected is ideal. The causative strain cannot be eliminated through these measures, but the situation can be kept workable.

This is not the case for rabbitries infected with the more virulent O15:H- (biotype 3) and, to a lesser extent, O103 (biotype 8) strains. They cannot be eliminated by treatment, and only extremely high doses of neomycin (1 g/litre) will lower mortality rates to an acceptable level. Healthy-looking carriers keep the infection going in the rabbitry and, when sold for breeding, infect other farms. 'Stamping out' should in fact be the prescribed remedy, although most rabbit breeders will object, since this measure itself causes high financial losses and because healthy animals to replace their breeding stock are so difficult to find. The high dosage of neomycin cannot be administered for a long period; it is sometimes prescribed to enable the owner to postpone the 'stamping out' procedure.

Clostridial enterotoxaemia

Occurrence. The natural disease occurs mostly in young animals 3-5 weeks old in all kinds of farms, but does not constitute an economical problem in most of them. It has been recorded in barrier-maintained colonies also, suggesting that the aetiological agent is ubiquitous.

Cause. Toxin-producing *Clostridium spiroforme*. Other *Clostridia* have also been isolated from rabbits, but so far there is no convincing evidence that they play an important role. The toxin produced by *C. spiroforme* closely resembles iota toxin, which is formed by *C. perfringens* type E.

Pathogenesis. There is both a spontaneous form and a form caused by administering antibiotics which are toxic for rabbits. In both cases rapid multiplication of the toxin-producing *C. spiroforme* is seen.

Symptoms. The spontaneous form always follows an acute course. Animals of any age above 3 weeks can become infected, though it is mostly those in the weaning age group of 3-6 weeks old that are affected. The disease may be endemic on an industrial rabbitry. Often more than one animal dies in each affected nest.

The form that results from the administration of antibiotics may be anything from acute (for example, with lincomycin) to chronic (for example, with broad-spectrum penicillin). The appetite falls off shortly after administration of the medicine. Death occurs some time from 2 days to 3 weeks later.

Lesions. The most noticeable lesion is the haemorrhagic inflammation of the caecum. There is often only a small amount of watery to mucoid, blood-coloured caecum contents. Some mucus may be found in the colon. If the animal died acutely, its nutritional condition will still be good and the liquid faeces found in the posterior end will not yet have dried up.

Diagnosis. This is based on symptoms and lesions. The method for confirming the presence of the toxin is difficult and expensive. Staining of caecal wall scrapings may reveal the presence of typical curled Gram-positive bacteria. They resemble horseshoes or pigtails (Plate 19). This is a useful aid in diagnosis.

Treatment. With the spontaneous form which takes an acute course, treatment of the individual animal always comes too late. With outbreaks, broad-spectrum antibiotics can be administered (for example, tetracycline, nitrofurantoins) but these cannot eradicate the disease. Enterotoxaemia is usually not a problem, since only sporadic cases are observed in most infected farms.

Prognosis is poor for rabbits which have become ill after administration of a toxic antibiotic. Only vancomycin is active as an antidote, but is too expensive to justify its use in rabbits. Other antibacterials such as potentiated sulphonamides and neomycin result only in minimal effects.

Tyzzer's disease

Occurrence. The disease occurs in many different animal species, but is most important in laboratory animal units. It is best known in rodents but is also found in rabbits raised for meat. Stress situations can cause acute outbreaks.

Cause. Bacillus piliformis, a motile Gram-negative spore-forming bacillus; it is an obligatory cell parasite, which means that it cannot be cultivated in inert environments.

Symptoms. With the acute course:
• Depression, watery diarrhoea, high mortality rate, especially among rabbits of weaning age.
With the chronic course:
• Chronic weight loss.

Lesions. In acute cases:
• Dehydration.

- Oedema of the intestinal wall, especially of the caecum.
- Necrosis of the mucosa of the caecum and proximal colon.
- Necrotic foci in the liver (up to 2 mm diameter) occur in a small percentage of affected animals, as opposed to rodents in which they are considered very typical.
- In some animals, degenerative lesions are found in the myocardium.

Chronic cases:

- Stenosis of the ileum is a characteristic sequel of the inflammation of the intestinal wall.

Diagnosis. Diagnosis of Tyzzer's disease is not easily made. The presence of intracellular bacilli should be demonstrated through histological examination of liver foci or in scrapings of the intestinal wall (ileum). They can be demonstrated with the Giemsa staining technique, or better with the Warthin–Starry silver impregnation technique which is expensive (the latter staining technique is not used for ileal wall scrapings). For this, rabbits showing acute symptoms of the disease that have just died or been sacrificed are needed. The bacteria cannot always be demonstrated, and certainly not in chronic cases. Often the typical lesions are all one has on which to base the diagnosis.

Treatment. All clinically sick animals have to be removed; do not attempt to treat them. Few antibiotics are active. Tetracyclines are administered on the basis of about half the normal dosage for a period of at least 1 month (250 ppm in the feed or 125 mg/litre water).

Prevention. Stress situations should be avoided, especially over-population. In case of an outbreak the evacuated batteries or compartments should be cleaned and disinfected.

Viral enteritis

So far there has been no clear proof that viruses play an aetiological role in the complex intestinal pathology of weaned rabbits. Rotavirus does occur in suckling rabbits, but it is not known whether it causes disease with significant economical importance; after experimental infection it produces only shortening of the intestinal villi.

Corona- and parvoviruses have also been isolated from the intestinal tracts of rabbits afflicted with diarrhoea, but experimental infections have yielded either dubious or negative results.

Parasitic intestinal disorders

Coccidiosis

In traditional rabbit keeping coccidiosis has been, and still is, one of the most important causes of sickness and death. Industrial rabbitries also are affected by coccidiosis, though on these it usually only results in retarded growth of the broiler rabbits. This development can be attributed to the better hygienic conditions attained with wire mesh floors and to the addition of coccidiostats in the pellets.

There are nine different *Eimeria* spp. which cause coccidiosis in rabbits; one causes liver coccidiosis while the others are intestinal.

Liver coccidiosis

Cause. Eimeria stiedae

Occurrence. On both traditional and industrial farms. When the disease is endemic only the young rabbits are affected. Older rabbits develop a strong immunity to *E. stiedae*, but not to the intestinal *Eimeria* spp. Coccidiostats are now commonly added to the feed, but the most frequently used coccidiostat, robenidin, which inhibits fully intestinal coccidiosis, lacks activity against *E. stiedae*. The situation was just the opposite when sulpha drug additives were still permitted in the feed pellets.

Symptoms. Retarded growth, though seldom death. The disease is most often only discovered at the time of slaughter.

Lesions. Moderately to very greatly enlarged liver (Plate 20). Presence in the liver of abscesses which range from small to the size of a pea. These lesions reduce the commercial value of the rabbits since the liver is inedible. This is the principal reason why the disease is treated on smaller farms.

Diagnosis. Microscopic examination of a drop of the gall bladder contents for the presence of *Eimeria stiedae* oöcysts.

Treatment. All the sulphonamides (see section on treatment of intestinal coccidiosis, below) are effective. Sulphaquinoxalin with or without diaveridin or aminopterin (so-called sulphonamide potentiators) is recommended.

Intestinal coccidiosis

Cause. As already noted, there are eight different *Eimeria* species which cause intestinal coccidiosis. The task of distinguishing all

Table 16.2 Properties of *Eimeria* spp. that cause intestinal coccidiosis in rabbits

Species	Localization	Pathogenicity	Lesions
E. coecicola	Ileum Caecum	Slight growth retardation	
E. flavescens	Caecum Colon	Anorexia Severe diarrhoea Weakness Weight loss Mortality	Thickening of the intestinal wall with pin-point haemorrhages in caecum and colon
E. intestinalis	Ileum Caecum	Same as *E.* *flavescens*	Greyish-white foci in ileum and ileo-caecal valve
E. irresidua	Small intestine	Only slight growth retardation	
E. magna	Ileum Caecum	Growth retardation Diarrhoea	White foci on the intestinal wall
E. media	Jejunum	Not well known: slight diarrhoea or obstipation	
E. perforans	Small intestine	Slight growth retardation	
E. piriformis (rare)	Caecum Colon	Mortalities	

these types from one another is the work of a specialist, though some of the sporulated oöcysts have such typical characteristics that, with a little practice, they can nevertheless be identified. These distinctions are of much importance since the different species vary greatly in their pathogenic effects. Table 16.2 presents some important characteristics of the eight types. Some of them, such as *E. flavescens* and *E. intestinalis*, are very pathogenic, producing high mortality after experimental infection with even relatively low doses. Others cause only slightly retarded growth which in practice will simply go unnoticed. *E. magna*, which causes serious diarrhoea and retarded growth, is easily recognized by the little collar, or wings, at the level of the micropyle. The non-pathogenic *E. perforans* can be distinguished by the absence of a micropyle and by its very small size (20 × 13 micrometers). The equally non-pathogenic *E. coecicola* is recognized by its oblong shape.

Symptoms. Depend on the type of *Eimeria* species involved.

Diagnosis. In practice it is usually not possible to identify the species (except for *E. magna*). The veterinarian must base his diagnosis on the number of oöcysts per microscopic field or per gram faeces and on the overall picture of symptoms and lesions. The OPG determination (oöcysts per gram faeces or intestinal contents) can be useful. The presence of only a few oöcysts does not rule out the diagnosis of 'coccidiosis' as the cause of death. However, it certainly does not confirm it, since practically all rabbits are more or less infected, unless they receive pellets with a coccidiostat.

Differential diagnosis. *Escherichia coli* enteritis and clostridial enterotoxaemia. When there are few oöcysts and these cannot be identified, then a differential diagnosis is extremely difficult without histological examination.

Treatment. Hygienic measures must be taken; otherwise none of the rest of the therapy makes any sense. Broiler rabbits should be housed on wire mesh rather than on straw. Certain wire cage systems are, however, less appropriate than others — especially the multilevel cages with transport belts for manure removal. The distance between the wire mesh and the manure is too small and the manure can spatter on the rabbits' paws. In addition, on such transport belts conditions are favourable for sporulation of the oöcysts. The same holds for scrape-off systems. Deep-pit systems are better in this respect, because in the deep layer of manure the conditions do not permit sporulation. For additional hygienic measures, see Chapter 6.

As for preventive treatment, most types of feed contain the very effective coccidiostat, robenidine. As noted above, robenidine is not sufficiently active against coccidiosis of the liver. Also, its effectiveness against intestinal coccidiosis can fall off with time when resistance develops.

Metichloropindol, another coccidiostatic compound, has long been the only one permitted under EEC regulations for use in rabbits, even though as early as 1970 it had already been proven that this product, in fact, was not effective with this animal species.

When an outbreak of coccidiosis occurs, a cure with sulphonamides is indicated, even when feed containing coccidiostat is already in use (see Chapter 22).

The treatment should take into account the possibility of reinfection. Thus a minimum of two periods of treatment are required. Good results are obtained with two periods of 7 days each, with a pause of 7 days in between.

Cryptosporidiosis

Sporadically, *Cryptosporidia* are seen during the histological examination of the intestinal lining of young broiler rabbits (4–6 weeks). Usually, though, they occur in association with other intestinal pathogens. The pathogenic significance of this parasite in weaned rabbits is unknown. In infant rabbits, they can cause serious growth retardation with only discrete and transitory diarrhoea.

Cryptosporidia can be detected in intestinal smears with the carbolfuchsine staining method described in Chapter 12.

Flagellates

On microscopic inspection, *Giardia* is sometimes found in the contents of the small intestine of rabbits which have just died or been killed and which have had diarrhoea. The significance of this observation in unknown. When no other cause is found, dimetridazole can be prescribed. This product appears also to be effective against some other forms of enteritis of unknown aetiology.

Liver fluke (rare in rabbits)

Fasciola hepatica occurs both in wild and in domesticated rabbits that eat grass from river banks or wet pasture land.

Symptoms. Cachexia, bad general condition, death.

Diagnosis. Demonstration of the parasite or its eggs at necropsy or during coprological examination.

Prevention. No feed grass should be taken from infected pasture land.

Tapeworms (rare)

Tapeworms are encountered only occasionally and almost only in wild rabbits.

Cysticercosis (common in 'backyard' rabbits)

Cause. Cysticercus pisiformis. The rabbit functions as intermediate host for one of the tapeworms found in dogs, *Taenia pisiformis.*

Lesions. The vesicles are located in the abdominal cavity, especially in the mesentery and to a lesser extent in the liver. These are almost always discovered at the time of slaughter, or during the necropsy after the rabbit has died of another disease (Plate 22). In exceptional cases, when widespread migratory lesions have formed in the liver after a very serious infection, a rabbit can die of cysticercosis.

Cysticercosis is seldom the cause of death, however, but is an indication of hygienic shortcomings. In these cases the search certainly must be carried on to find other parasites.

Prevention. Eliminate contact between dogs and rabbits; never feed dogs the entrails of rabbits.

Trichostrongylidae

Various species occur, but only when greens or grass is used for feed, and thus not in industrial rabbitries.

Graphidium strigosum, the stomach worm, is common among wild rabbits and regularly appears in domestic ones. The small worms (1–2 cm) are red and are found on the mucous membrane of the stomach (Plate 23). It causes weight loss and even death.

There are also a few species that occur in the small intestine. Only *Trichostrongylus retortaeformis* is found regularly in Europe. Very rarely, this one can occur in rabbits kept on wire mesh.

Treatment. All benzimidazole derivates (see Chapter 22).

Oxyuridae

Only *Passalurus ambiguus* is very common, and this is the case with battery rabbits as well as with traditionally kept animals. These worms are about 0.5 cm long and can be massively present in the caecum. It is doubtful whether they are pathogenic.

Intestinal disorders of unknown aetiology

Mucoid enteropathy (constipation; caecal impaction; gut stasis)

With various intestinal conditions the presence of a thick, gelatinous lump or mucus in the colon is such a noticeable phenomenon that in earlier times it seemed only natural to call the condition 'mucoid enteritis'. This mucus, however, occurs with various forms of enteritis, for example, with antibiotic-induced enterotoxaemia. The phenomenon is probably a reaction to slowed intestinal flow or to non-specific irritation. At present we apply the term 'mucoid enteropathy' only to one particular affection. Since one of its characteristics is the absence of inflammatory lesions, the term 'mucoid enteritis' has also been rejected and replaced by 'mucoid enteropathy'. As constipation of the caecum is a frequent symptom, the terms 'caecal impaction', and 'constipation' can be considered also as appropriate.

Aetiology. Unknown. A condition very similar to this mucoid enteropathy can be induced artificially by ligating the caecum, thus suggesting that the obstipation is at the origin. Still, however, the reason why rabbits get obstipated and the way the other symptoms develop are not known.

Other evidence suggests that the disease is contagious, and probably of bacterial origin.

Occurrence. Most often in rabbits 2 weeks after weaning. Those which show the highest weight gain seem to be more frequently affected.

Symptoms. Acute to subacute. The rabbits languish for a few days, but this stage may pass unnoticed. They sit apart from the others; they stop eating but drink a lot; they may grind their teeth as an expression of pain and keep the stomach pulled in. By palpation a hard core, the impacted caecum, is usually located in the right side of the abdominal cavity. Shortly before death, fluid runs out of the nose and mouth and there are signs of breathing difficulties. The mortality rate can reach 60–100% in this age group.

Lesions. The stomach is overfull with watery contents. The small intestine ranges from normal to overly full, without inflammation. The contents of the caecum are either dried up (Plate 24) or just a little too watery. In most instances, the first 5–10 cm of the colon contains a dried up mass; further on a tough lump of mucus may be found. In 60% of the cases there is a very typical pneumonia with redness of the apical lobes. The borderline between inflamed and healthy lung tissue is sharply demarcated. In the trachea a spumous fluid is sometimes found. With histological examination, foreign bodies (plant cells) are detected in the bronchi and even deep in the lung tissue (see Chapter 15).

Treatment. Curative: The following curative treatment has been recommended: 250mg metamizole with 2.5mg methindizate hydrochloride (Isaverin, Bayer) and 1mg dexamethasone sodium phosphate (Dexadreson, Intervet) should be given intramuscularly.

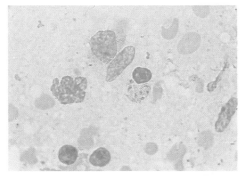

Plate 1. Old French lop doe with well developed dewlap. This is a normal condition in old rabbits, especially in females of heavy breeds.

Plate 2. May Grünwald–Giemsa staining of liver impression smear. Banana–shaped *Toxoplasma* tachyzoids are visible in the centre of the preparation.

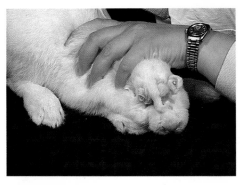

Plate 3. Multiple subcutaneous abscesses, which resulted in deformation of the head. *Pasteurella multocida* was isolated in pure cultures from the lesions.

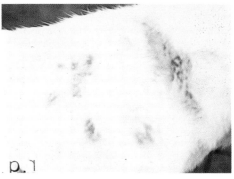

Plate 4. Mastitis caused by rabbit specific *Staphylococcus aureus*: superficial purulent dermatitis round the teats.

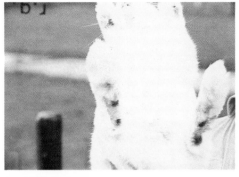

Plate 5. Ulcerative pododermatitis; all four paws are affected. Such cases are often encountered on farms which are infected with rabbit pathogenic *Staphylococcus aureus*.

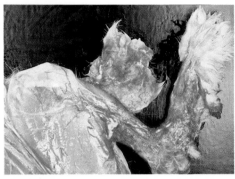

Plate 6. Lymphangitis secondary to chronic 'sore hocks' infected with *Staphylococcus aureus*.

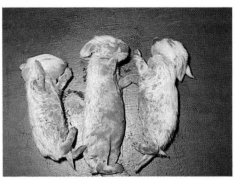

Plate 7. Three suckling rabbits (about 10 days old) from a litter which died out completely with cutaneous staphyloccosis. They show a typical exudative dermatitis: the skin is wet and seeded with superficial pustules.

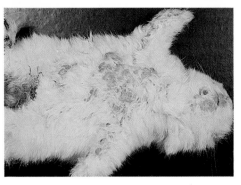

Plate 8. Cutaneous staphylococcosis: subcutaneous abscesses in a 3 week old rabbit.

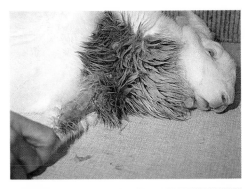

Plate 9. Moist dermatitis, infected with *Pseudomonas aeruginosa*. In this case the skin shows partial alopecia and the pus colours the fur with a typical blue-green pigment. This striking characteristic is not always seen with *Pseudomonas* skin infections.

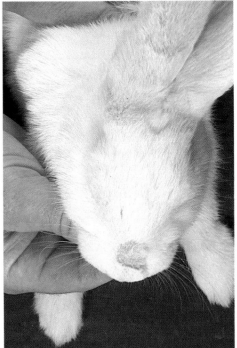

Plate 10. Ringworm caused by *Microsporum canis*: partial alopecia on the nose.

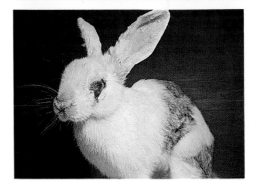

Plate 11. Myxomatosis, acute form. Swelling of the head and purulent blepharoconjunctivitis are typical.

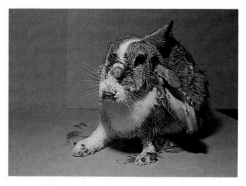

Plate 12. Myxomatosis, nodular form. Multiple, well defined myxoma are present on the ears, head and forepaws.

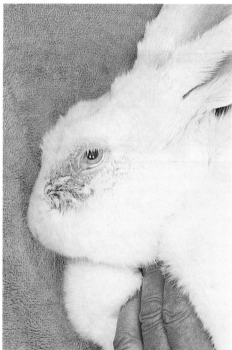

Plate 13. Chronic conjunctivitis in a rabbit; alopecia down the medial eye corner.

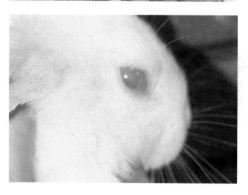

Plate 14. Hereditary glaucoma in a 6 week old rabbit.

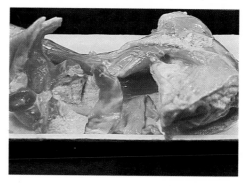

Plate 15. Rabbit carcass, ready for consumption. After opening of the chest cavity, it appeared to be filled with pus. *Pasteurella multocida* is the cause of such purulent pleuropneumonia.

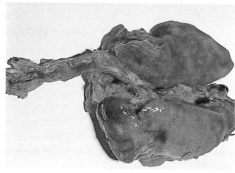

Plate 16. Acute pleuropneumonia caused by virulent strains of *Pasteurella multocida*. Lungs are congested and covered with a fibrinous layer. Haemorrhagic fluid is seen in the trachea.

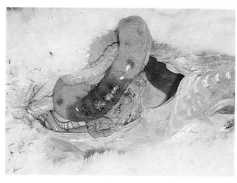

Plate 17. Subserosal bleedings on the caecal wall of a rabbit which died from coli-diarrhoea. Such haemorrhages are only present in a restricted number of cases and most often look like 'paint brush' bleedings.

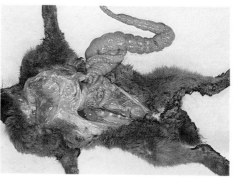

Plate 18. Typical necropsy picture of a rabbit dead from coli-diarrhoea. In this case the appearance of the caecal wall is only hyperaemic and oedematous. Its contents are light brown, bad smelling and fluid.

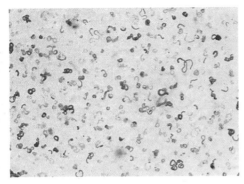

Plate 19. *Clostridium spiroforme*, after cultivation. They appear as relatively long, curled rods. These consist in fact of a chain of several semi-circular smaller rods.

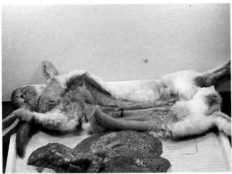

Plate 20. *Eimeria stiedae* infection. The liver is enlarged and seeded with multiple abscesses. Usually the complaint does not take such an acute course and causes only growth retardation.

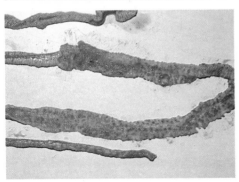

Plate 21. Intestinal coccidiosis, which resulted in a chronic inflammation of the small intestine.

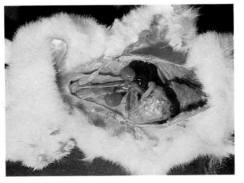

Plate 22. *Cysticercus pisiformis* vesicles on the mesentery of a rabbit.

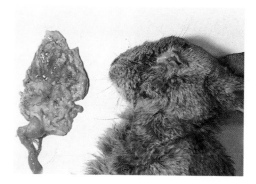

Plate 23. *Graphidium strigosum* is a stomach worm which appears as small red filaments attached to the inner wall of the stomach.

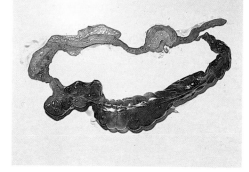

Plate 24. Caecal impaction–mucoid enteropathy complex: caecum and colon. The caecal contents are dried and mixed with gas; the colon contains a lump of tenacious mucus.

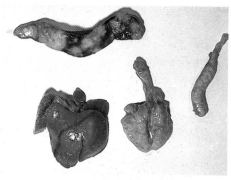

Plate 25. Appendix (right), lungs (bottom middle), liver (bottom left) and spleen (top) of a rabbit which died of rodentiosis. Note the necrotic foci in the liver, spleen and wall of the appendix and the enlargement of the spleen.

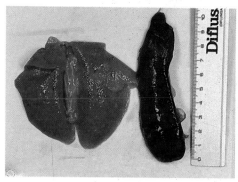

Plate 26. *Toxoplasma gondii* infection. Congestion of the lungs and enlargement of the spleen, which can attain about ten times its normal volume.

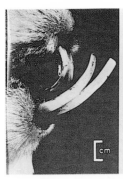
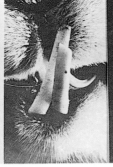

Plate 27. Malocclusion of the incisors, which results in dental overgrowth. The uppers are curved inwards, while the lowers are more straight and easily visible without opening the mouth.

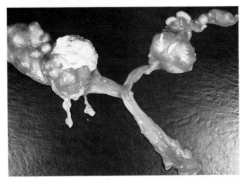

Plate 28. Purulent metritis: multiple abscesses have developed. Such a lesion is often caused by *Staphylococcus aureus*.

Preventive: Tetracyclines (250 mg/l drinking water or 500 ppm in the feed) are very effective. If, for an extended period, all the young are treated for 10 days after weaning, the disease may totally disappear. This usually cannot be done via the drinking water since the young of all ages are housed together. Instead, so-called medicinal weaning feeds containing antibiotics can be used; this is common practice in France. When these animals go to slaughter there are no problems with residual antibiotics.

Intestinal paresis in does

Occurrence. End of pregnancy or during lactation. Primiparous does are more often affected than multiparous. Mortalities among does in production are recorded in small-scale as well as in large-scale rabbitries.

Cause. Unknown. Pregnancy toxaemia is suspected, or else hypocalcaemia in lactating animals. These terms suggest the existence of metabolic disorders in highly productive rabbits, which have in fact not yet been convincingly demonstrated.

Symptoms. Anorexia, abdominal distension, rapid death. Weakness of the muscles or paralysis is observed only in exceptional cases.

Lesions. Overfilling of the whole intestinal system. Most often the liver shows fatty degeneration. A large mass of gelatinous mucus may be present in the colon. There are no inflammatory lesions in the intestinal tract. The necropsy picture suggests that the affection is very similar to mucoid enteropathy in broiler rabbits.

Prognosis. Poor. As the disease usually takes a hyperacute course and most animals are found dead without previously showing any symptoms, treatment usually comes too late.

Treatment. No effective treatment is known. With animals that show muscle weakness or paralysis, the administration of calcium preparations, intended for use in cows, can be tried. When their young are more than 3 weeks old, they can be weaned, which will also increase the chances of survival of the dam. Others suggest that the administration of cortisone will help.

As the affection is similar to mucoid enteropathy, a symptomatic treatment against colic signs could be tried: 250 mg metamizole with 2.5 mg methindizate (Isaverin, Bayer) together with 1 mg dexamethasone sodium phosphate (Dexadreson, Intervet), administered by intramuscular injection.

Other causes of disorders or lesions in the intestinal system

Dental aberrations

See Chapter 20.

Oral papillomatosis

This condition has only been diagnosed in North America, in *Oryctolagus* as well as in *Sylvilagus*. Small (1–2 mm) sessile or pedunculated white nodules are found in the mouth cavity, usually on the ventral surface of the tongue. No harmful effects have been recorded. A similar disease has once been described in the United Kingdom, in a laboratory unit. This affection was somewhat different because the polyps were not located at the same site but merely on the gum behind and around the lower incisor teeth. The cause is a papilloma virus which differs from the Shope cutaneous papilloma virus.

Trichobezoars in the stomach

See section on self-plucking of wool in Chapter 13.

Toxoplasmosis

With acute toxoplasmosis, catarrhal enteritis is also observed (see Chapter 19).

Peritonitis

Besides being a result of either stomach rupture or trauma, peritonitis can also be a form of acute pasteurellosis (see Chapter 19), or of staphylococcosis (see section on Cutaneous staphylococcosis in Chapter 13 and also Chapter 19).

Rodentiosis and salmonellosis

Small white foci on the appendix and the sacculus rotundus (see Chapter 19).

17 / Diseases of the urogenital system

External sexual organs

Myxomatosis

The pseudo-tumours that accompany myxomatosis have a predilection for the peri-anal region (see Chapter 13).

Spirochaetosis (treponematosis; rabbit syphilis)

Cause

Treponema cuniculi. This germ is clearly different from *Treponema pallidum* which causes a venereal disease in humans. The two diseases have no connection with one another.

Occurrence

Extremely rare. Non-existent in industrial situations.

Lesions and symptoms

The general condition of the animal remains good, because metastasis to the internal organs does not occur. The lesions on the external sex organs begin as redness or oedema, then vesicles appear and later brown scabs form from the exudate. The epithelium ulcerates. Apparently the lesions are painful. On the head, skin lesions appear, especially around the muzzle, as a sequel of auto-inoculation. Most cases heal, though some remain asymptomatic carriers.

Diagnosis

1 Dark field microscopy of scrapings from the lesions.
2 Histology: silver dye.
3 Serological tests: only performed in specialized laboratories.

Differential diagnosis

Healed nodular myxomatosis also produces scabs.

Treatment

Antibiotics: tetracyclines, chloramphenicol.

Penicillin, which is the antibiotic of choice in humans for spirochaetosis, is not recommended for rabbits because toxicity in this animal species has been reported; broad-spectrum penicillins are very toxic (see Chapter 22).

Diseases of the kidneys

Nephritis

At necropsy, macroscopically visible kidney lesions are not frequently seen. Possible necropsy findings include: irregular grey patches (nosemosis), scars (nosemosis), infarcts (staphylococcosis, human strains), calcification (in older rabbits) and pyelonephritis (staphylococcosis, pasteurellosis).

Histological examinations, however, reveal that kidney disease is as common as in other animal species. No data are available on the occurrence of clinical sequellae of renal failure in older animals, but it is very likely that such symptoms exist.

Diseases of the bladder

Urolithiasis

White precipitates in the bladder are normal and do not indicate inflammation of the bladder; they consist of amorphous calcium carbonate crystals. Urolithiases in male rabbits has been reported. We have found bladder stones in dwarf rabbits of related origins. Problems arise when the stones become lodged in the exit from the bladder or in the urethra.

Symptoms. Continual straining of the abdomen, sucked-in stomach, gnashing teeth. Caution: the straining is often not recognized, but considered a respiratory symptom or a nervous disturbance. When the stones are moving free in the bladder, an animal can show attacks of such symptoms at irregular time intervals.

Diagnosis. Radiography.

Prognosis. Depends on the general condition, which is usually very bad.

Treatment. Surgical removal of the stone can be attempted in pet rabbits.

Metritis
See Chapter 21.

Orchitis-epididymitis
See Chapter 21.

18 / Disorders of the nervous system and related conditions

Paralysis

Coccidiosis

Some rabbits severely affected by coccidiosis show signs of paralysis, especially in the hind paws.

Fractured lumbar vertebrae (broken back, dislocation of lumbar vertebrae)

This often occurs, also with pet rabbits. Possible causes include wrong handling, a fall, suddenly hopping in the cage, etc. The anamnesis is often difficult, in which case it is impossible to find the actual cause.

Cause. The spinal column of the rabbit is not very flexible and when stressed breaks at the weakest place, most often the seventh lumbar vertebra. In some cases there is only dislocation of vertebrae.

Symptoms. Paralysis in the hindquarters. When the spinal marrow has been injured, there is also incontinence: the hindquarters are soiled with urine and droppings.

Diagnosis. Radiography.

Prognosis. Poor in the case of serious damage of the spinal cord, when the animal has lost control of voiding of urine and defaecation. In other cases, the backbone can heal enough to enable the animal to move, and pets should not always be destroyed.

Treatment. Depends on the severity of the lesions. In most cases euthanasia is recommended. Does with small young can be left for a few days until the young are old enough (see section on Raising motherless young, Chapter 21).

Other causes of paralysis

These exist, but are difficult to establish. Lactating does can show paralysis and muscle weakness at about 3 weeks post-partum; hypocalcaemia is supposed to be at the origin (see section on Intestinal paresis in does, Chapter 16). Listeriosis produces paralysis or other nervous symptoms only in exceptional cases.

78

On one occasion on a large industrial rabbitry, we observed an outbreak of a disease consisting mainly of nervous disorders. This occurred after a change in feed. Histological examination revealed a non-purulent encephalitis, which suggested a viral cause. No viruses were found, however, and experimental infection by inoculating SPF rabbits proved unsuccessful.

Borna's disease has been described in the literature as a cause of encephalitis in rabbits, referring to cases occurring in Central Europe only. In addition, paralysis has been observed in connection with chronic toxoplasmosis (diagnosis: serological examination or post-mortem histology). Encephalitozoonosis (nosemosis) can also cause paralysis.

Rabbits suffering from pyometra are unwilling to move and show stiffness of the hind legs. It is unclear if these symptoms have a central origin or are simply a reaction to abdominal pain.

Rabies

Rabbits are subject to this disease, but actual cases are extremely rare, even in European regions where the disease is endemic among the foxes. Rabies should be suspected only when wild rabbits from infected regions show nervous symptoms. Take protective measures when handling such rabbits.

Epilepsy

Epilepsy occurs in white rabbit breeds that have white fur and blue eyes, such as Beveren white and Vienna white. The animal can succumb during a convulsion. No specific lesions are found post-mortem, though the cause of death can be surmised from the anamnesis and from the unphysiological position in which the dead animal is found.

Torticollis (wry neck)

Causes. Torticollis and rolling movements frequently occur with infection of the middle ear by weakly virulent strains of *P. multocida*. Rhinitis and snuffles do not always accompany such symptoms (see also section on Snuffles, Chapter 15). In serious cases the animal is no longer able to eat or drink.

Other cases have been reported in the literature, in which no exudate was found upon dissection of the bulla tympanica. It was assumed that *Nosema cuniculi* was the cause of the disease. Note: such symptoms have no connection with ear mange.

Lesions. Presence of pus in the bulla tympanica.

Prognosis. Poor for the individual animal. Only rarely will antibiotics make the symptoms disappear.

Nosemosis

Cause and occurrence. Nosema cuniculi (= Encephalitozoon cuniculi). This parasite is very common, but the disease remains practically always latent. It is mainly a problem in laboratory rabbits.

Symptoms. All sorts of nervous disorders, including convulsions, torticollis and paralysis.

Lesions. Kidney lesions: small, sunken areas on the surface of the kidney, or multiple pinhead-sized white spots and scars.

The lesions in the central nervous system are microscopic: granulomatous encephalitis is the characteristic lesion. The parasites cannot always be demonstrated in histological preparations.

Diagnosis. It is difficult to determine if a rabbit is infected with *Encephalitozoon*; only specialized laboratories are able to perform the necessary investigations. This can be important for laboratory animal units, because nosemosis can disturb many neurological experiments. Different serological tests have been developed for this purpose (immunofluorescence, India ink immuno-technique and indirect micro-haemagglutination test).

In rabbits with typical symptoms the diagnosis can be made by histological examination. The parasites cannot always be demonstrated but the typical granulomatous lesions are considered sufficient for proof.

Treatment. No effective treatment is known. Besides, in the individual animal the disease is only discovered at post-mortem examination.

Splay leg

See Chapter 20.

19 / Systemic diseases

Rodentiosis

Cause. Yersinia pseudotuberculosis. This bacterium is also very pathogenic for birds and guinea pigs. Rats and mice function as carriers.

Occurrence. Not in industrial rabbitries. It is most often diagnosed in the winter, in small units where rodents have access to the cages or the feed.

Symptoms. Not specific. Poor general condition, progressive weight loss.

Lesions. Very typical. Cachexia, moderate to great enlargement of spleen with necrotic foci, multiple necrotic foci at the level of Sacculus rotundus and appendix. These necrotic foci are localized at the transition ileum–caecum, and at the top of the caecum (Plate 25). Lymphoid tissue is concentrated at these sites (see Fig. 3.2).

Diagnosis. Bacteriological examination of the necrotic foci. The diagnosis cannot be established in an animal that is still alive.

Differential diagnosis. Salmonellosis and toxoplasmosis.

Treatment. Low doses of nitrofurantoin (100–200 mg/l) or chloramphenicol (100 mg/l) are given for prolonged periods (3 weeks or 1 month).

Prevention. Rodent control.

Salmonellosis

Occurrence. Rabbits seldom contract this disease, though they are susceptible to it. Salmonellosis almost only occurs in small units of rabbits housed in unhygienic conditions. Exceptional cases have been attributed to contaminated feed.

Cause. Usually *Salmonella typhimurium*, though other *Salmonella* serotypes may be involved.

Symptoms. Depression, fever, and sometimes but not always diarrhoea. High mortality rate along with abortion by pregnant does.

Lesions. Hyperacute form: Septicaemic lesions; congestion of the organs, pinpoint haemorrhages.

Acute form: The most noticeable lesion is the greatly swollen spleen, which can be about 10 times its normal volume. Necrotic foci may be found in the spleen, as well as in the liver and on the Peyer's patches, Sacculus rotundus and appendix, as with rodentiosis. Metritis is found in does that are pregnant or have aborted.

Diagnosis. Bacteriological examination.

Treatment: Curative treatment is seldom recommended, since treated animals may become asymptomatic carriers.

Prevention. Hygienic measures. Trace the source of infection, which can, for example, be the feed or rodents . . . but this is no easy task. Remove feed and straw; thoroughly clean and disinfect cages.

Acute pasteurellosis (haemorrhagic septicaemia)

See also section on Snuffles, Chapter 15.

Cause. Certain highly virulent strains of *Pasteurella multocida.* There is no clear distinction between those strains that are high and those that are low in virulence; the rabbit Pasteurellae form rather a continuous spectrum in this regard.

Occurrence. Mainly among rabbits housed in small units. Rabbits that are either carriers or have been in contact with the lesser virulent pasteurellae (typical 'snuffles' pasteurellae) are no longer sensitive to highly virulent strains. This is probably the reason why these highly virulent strains seldom cause disease on the large rabbitries, which are almost always infected with the weakly virulent strains.

Symptoms. With certain strains mortality is hyperacute, within 24 hours after experimental infection. Such strains are also pathogenic for fowl but very seldom occur. With most other strains, symptoms include purulent discharge from the nose, acute dyspnoea and rapid death (within 4–7 days after experimental infection).

Lesions. Hyperacute form: lung congestion, scattered haemorrhages, haemorrhagic tracheitis.

Acute form: same, but also purulent or fibrous pneumonia, pericarditis and/or peritonitis.

Diagnosis. Bacteriological examination of the heart blood or bone marrow of a recently dead animal. May–Grünwald–Giemsa staining of a bloodsmear or an impression smear of the trachea will sometimes make bipolar bacteria visible, though only in the hyperacute form.

Treatment. Treatment with antibiotics usually comes too late for the individual animal. The rest of the animals in the shed can be treated with antibiotics.

Prevention. Vaccination with inactivated vaccines produces very good results. See section on Snuffles, Chapter 15.

Toxoplasmosis

Cause. Toxoplasma gondii. After a proliferation phase with rapid intracellular development of tachyzoids, a rest phase sets in, during which cysts appear in the tissue. Usually this phase remains latent in the animal. The proliferation phase can result in serious illness in rabbits, with high mortality.

Occurrence. There is a high level of seroprevalence. Seropositive rabbits have cysts in their tissues and most of them remain healthy.

In some circumstances a true epidemic takes place, with an especially high incidence of illness and death among pregnant and nursing does.

The source of infection for toxoplasmosis in rabbits is feed contaminated by cat faeces which contain oöcysts. As rabbits are herbivores, rodents cannot infect them since they do not excrete oöcysts.

Symptoms. Acute form: anorexia, listlessness, fever, death after a few days. Morbidity is highest with pregnant or lactating does.

Chronic form: remains almost always asymptomatic. Occasionally central nervous symptoms may be seen.

Lesions. In rabbits which have died from the acute form, the following lesions are observed: congestion of the organs, inflammatory lesions in the lungs, swelling of the liver. Most noticeable is the swelling of the spleen up to about 10 times its normal size (Plate 26).

Diagnosis. Not always easy. In the acute form tachyzoids can be seen in impression smears from the spleen and especially from the liver stained by the May–Grünwald–Giemsa technique, and also in histological sections. These tachyzoids die out quickly after the death of the host, however, so that a few hours later they can no longer be found. Another method of diagnosis is isolation in mice through intraperitoneal injection of a suspension prepared from spleen and liver tissue. The serological test (Sabin–Feldmann test) can be useful for the diagnosis of chronic toxoplasmosis.

Treatment. Potentiated sulphonamides can be tried.

Prevention. Avoid contamination. Possible sources of infection: fresh greens, straw or pellets contaminated with cat dung.

Zoonotic importance. Rabbits which either have, or have had, toxoplasmosis seldom constitute a danger for humans because the cysts in their tissues have little resistance to heat, and rabbit meat is well cooked and not intended to beaten raw. Direct handling can present some danger. Animals other than cats do not transmit the disease during the acute phase. The rabbit is important, however, as a reservoir which keeps the cycle alive.

Listeriosis

Cause. Listeria monocytogenes. Although this bacterium is ubiquitous, it seldom causes illness in rabbits.

Occurrence. In small units. Listeriosis is not a problem in industrial situations. The disease is most often diagnosed in wintertime.

Symptoms. Especially pregnant does or animals under stress (from inadequate feeding, for example) become sick. The symptoms are non-specific: depression, anorexia, death. Pregnant does may abort. Nervous disorders are seldom observed in rabbits, by contrast with other species.

Lesions. With acute septicaemia: congestion, pinpoint haemorrhages, oedema of the cervical and mesenteric lymph glands, serous fluid in the body cavities, necrotic foci in the liver and sometimes also in the spleen. Especially: purulent metritis in pregnant does; also dead fetuses in the uterus, unless already aborted.

Diagnosis. Bacteriological examination of the contents of the uterus, of the aborted fetuses, or of the liver or other organs of animals which have died from septicaemia.

Treatment. Tetracyclines are effective.

Tularaemia

Cause. Francisella tularensis. This bacterium can only be isolated on special media.

Occurrence. Francisella tularensis causes acute septicaemical illness in many vertebrates, including human beings. The infection is conveyed by insect bites or through handling of infected meat. There have been reports of epidemics in several States in the US involving the local cottontail rabbits, and in Norway involving a local species of hare; each instance was accompanied by a high number of cases in humans after the handling of rabbits or hares, or after insect bites. *Francisella* is able to invade the conjunctiva and the intact skin.

In Western and Southern Europe, tularaemia has only once been reported in wild *Oryctolagus* and never in domestic rabbits.

Staphylococcosis

Septicaemic forms of staphylococcosis are caused both by special rabbit pathogenic strains of *Staphylococcus aureus*, which principally result in a skin infection, and by strains of human origin. These human strains can produce abscesses and are important as secondary invaders of wounds in the paws (see section on sore hocks, Chapter 13). Septicaemia caused by human strains is a matter of sporadic cases, in contrast to the disease occasioned by the special rabbit pathogenic strains. Various lesions are observed after spreading in the internal organs. Pneumonia develops very often (see Chapter 15). Infarct formation in the kidneys is a very typical lesion, though we have only observed it with infection by human staphylococci. These lesions are irregular grey patches which are sunken in the centre. The delineation of diseased and healthy kidney tissue is sharp and red coloured.

Diagnosis. Isolation of the *S. aureus* in serious outbreaks, to be followed by biotyping and phagetyping of the isolated strains.

20 / Inherited conditions

Lethal defects

Certain rare conditions are now and then found among rabbits which are either born dead or have died shortly after birth: for example, hydrocephalus externus and spina bifida.

Sublethal defects

Dental aberrations

Dental overgrowth (mandibular prognathism, malocclusion of the incisors)

Malocclusion of the incisors is very common among all rabbit breeds. Mandibular prognathism (the mandibula being too long in relation to the maxilla) has a fatal outcome in nature because of the unusual arrangement of the teeth in lagomorphs.

The dental formula is: I(2/1); C(0/0); PM (3/2); M(3/3).

The four upper incisors are not lined up in a row, but are arranged in pairs, each with one tooth behind the other. The lagomorphs (rabbits and hares) differ from the rodents on this point. The back teeth, called peg teeth, are small and may be missing; in fact they are not needed by the animal. With the true incisors, both the upper and the lower, the layer of enamel is irregular in thickness: very thick in front, and virtually undeveloped on the back side. These incisors continue growing during the whole lifetime, the lower at the rate of 2.4 mm per week.

With normal teeth, the lower and upper incisors match and thus continuously wear each other down. Because of the hard enamel layer they wear less quickly in front than at the back and thus maintain a very sharp cutting edge.

When the teeth are abnormally positioned, which in most cases will be an inherited defect, the uppers and lowers no longer meet and thus no longer wear each other down, but simply keep growing longer and longer. When this defect is minimal it can be corrected in the early stages, because the lower incisors do not rest on the peg teeth, but on the upper front incisors. As the rabbit grows, the lower teeth move further forward until the grinding action is no longer possible. Thus it is possible that this defect, though innate, may not come to expression till the rabbit is older.

In rabbits that show dental overgrowth, the upper incisors curve sharply inward while the lowers grow in a broader curve outward (Plate 27). The lower teeth are readily visible upon general inspection, even without opening the mouth. Food intake gradually becomes impossible and the animals progressively lose weight.

Treatment. Trimming. The upper and lower incisors can easily be trimmed without sedation of the animal. Trimming should be repeated every 4–5 weeks, and many rabbit owners are able to do this themselves. Such treatment is only advised for pet rabbits; breeders of show rabbits should be warned that the condition is hereditary.

Malocclusion of the molars

This condition is much less common and, like malocclusion of the incisors, is in most cases hereditary. In rabbits the molars also grow continuously, though much more slowly than the incisors. When the lower jaw is too narrow, sharp points form on the molars. The points that form on the lower jaw injure the tongue, while those that form on the upper jaw produce lesions on the inner surface of the cheeks. Either abscesses of the tongue or necrosis of the tongue may develop. Continuous wetting of the dewlap may cause a condition called 'moist dermatitis'.

Symptoms. Difficulties with swallowing, hypersalivation, refusal of food (especially hard food), progressive weight loss.

Diagnosis. Not so easy as with overgrowth of the incisors, because the mouth opening of a rabbit is too small to permit thorough inspection of the mouth cavity; an otoscope should be used. Sedation is often necessary. Radiography can also be useful.

Prognosis. Poor, since the original defect cannot be eliminated and the trimming should be repeated at regular times. Since this intervention requires sedation or anaesthaesia, treatment is usually not recommended.

Treatment. In theory, regular filing or trimming would solve the problem.

Splay leg

'Splay leg' is the name used for the condition where rabbits cannot hold one or more paws in the normal position, but rather keep them spread. The defect can occur both in the fore- and hindpaws, or simultaneously in all four.

The phenomenon is not a matter of one single condition; rather it can be occasioned by various sorts of conditions such as hereditary luxation or subluxation of the femur, or hereditary nervous disorders. Such defects become expressed only when the rabbits leave the nest, or even later. 'Splay leg' is very common among fryer rabbits on industrial rabbitries, and especially among fryers from very small litters (one or two young). It is supposed that the quality of the floor of the nest box and of the straw is important; it should not be too smooth. It is also supposed that the weight of the young rabbits is the decisive factor: young from small nests are very heavy when they leave the nest.

Affected rabbits can move themselves over short distances, and so they easily manage to fatten themselves along with the rest of the group.

Again, breeders should be advised of the hereditary character of the defect.

Defects of the eyelids

See Chapter 14.

Glaucoma

See Chapter 14.

Other hereditary conditions, without detrimental effects

Yellow fat

The body fat of a rabbit is normally white. In some rabbit breeds a number of animals appear to have yellow fat; this is only observed when they are slaughtered.

This is caused by the absence of an enzyme which breaks down xanthophyll. Xanthophyll refers to a group of plant pigments which can function as provitamin A. The degree of discoloration depends on the amount of xanthophyll present in the feed, and can vary from light yellow to orange. The genetic factor is recessive.

The phenomenon has no negative effect on either health or productivity of the animal, but the characteristic is undesirable in broiler rabbits.

Serum atropinesterase

About 60% of the rabbits possess in their serum an enzyme which breaks down atropine. This does not affect their health; on the contrary such rabbits can even survive on a diet of belladonna leaves. But the presence or absence of the factor determines how the animal will react if atropine is administered, by injection or topically. This cannot be predicted.

21 / Breeding problems

Losses among sucklings

The losses from death previous to weaning on industrial rabbitries are very high compared with other animals. In France the mortality rate has been calculated to be 26.7% from birth to slaughter age, of which 18.9% occurs before weaning.

Dead kits individually represent little value, so the raiser usually remains unconcerned about this fact. In reality, the financial loss due to deaths previous to weaning is much more significant than that due, for example, to enzootic pneumonia. This is also the case on rabbitries which experience no trouble with diseases that specifically affect the neonates.

Above all, the fact that whole litters often are born dead or die soon after birth in industrial rabbitries constitutes a considerable problem. Nothing is known about the cause of the high number of dead neonati; the observed lesions are not specific and pathogenic bacteria are not isolated. It has been noted that some does never lose any kits at birth, while others have several deadborn young at each litter. Probably something similar is also the case with the bucks: it occurs more often with the progeny of some of them.

Possible causes of abortion and premature birth

Listeriosis and salmonellosis

See Chapter 19. Both diseases occur almost exclusively in small units and are rare.

Deaths among the neonati

Hereditary defects

See Chapter 20. The actual number is negligible.

Defective nesting behaviour

This is a phenomenon that may cause serious losses. The does may construct poor quality nests by plucking too little wool, or they may make their nest on the wire mesh floor rather than in the intended nest box. Some does are cannibalistic, and eat their young wholly or partially. Another phenomenon is nest watering: the does deposit their droppings and urine on the place where they have built their nest.

This behaviour can be caused by various factors:
• During the seasonally conditioned infertility period (see below) the percentages of neglect and cannibalism increase. This suggests that a hormonal factor plays a role.
• Mothering characteristics are partially inherited. Thus with hybrid rabbits importance is attached to breeding a good maternal instinct into the mother line. This should be taken into account on rabbitries which raise their own breeding stock.
• Housing and management. These problems almost never appear with pet or show rabbits which are kept on straw, except for nest watering, which appears often enough with these types. In wire cages, various sorts of nest boxes are used. The dimensions should not be too large, or the doe sometimes lies in it herself because it is more comfortable. Dimensions of 30 × 30 cm are sufficient. Does also like to build their nests at a deeper level, preferably in the dark. Our own experience has been that small, enclosed nest boxes hung on the cage with the floor 10 cm lower than that of the rest of the cage function very well compared with the roomier open-top wooden nest boxes that are placed inside the cage.

If large numbers of does refuse to have their litter in the intended place, the raiser should be advised to keep a close eye on the does during the period shortly before littering. If they appear to start building their nest on the wire mesh, he or she can lay a small board on the spot. After littering, the board is placed in the nest box. This makeshift will significantly reduce the losses, though it can only be employed in small units since it is so labour intensive.

To prevent nest watering, nest boxes that can be closed off from the rest of the cage should be used. The doe is placed in the maternity cage as soon as the pregnancy diagnosis is positive (12 days after breeding), but is not given access to the nest box until a few days before littering (gestation lasts 30–32 days). Meanwhile she will have chosen another place to urinate and to leave droppings.

Hypothermia

Being naked, newborn rabbits are very sensitive to cold. When born on
the wire mesh floor, they will die of hypothermia within a few hours.

At normal shed temperatures (12–16°C) no problems arise. The
nest temperature will be high enough if sufficient nest material is
provided, and if the doe plucks enough wool.

Note: the hay and straw is often eaten up by the doe within a few
days.

There can be problems when the weather gets cold if the shed is
not heated enough. In this case, a roomy wooden nest box is needed
since wood is insulating, and an extra thick layer of straw should be
provided. With such an arrangement, selected robust rabbits will
continue breeding in wire cages, even in unheated sheds and
freezing weather.

Diseases that specifically affect the neonates

As mentioned above, the death rate among newborn rabbits is always
relatively high. When sudden, abnormally high death rates are noted,
the cause may be cutaneous staphylococcosis (see Chapter 13) or
neonatal coli-diarrhoea (see Chapter 16). In either case, the kits are
found wet. With staphylococcosis, the skin is seeded with superficial
pustules. With coli-diarrhoea the young diffuse a bad odour and they
are wetted with a yellow fluid, though this may not be so obvious with
rabbit breeds that are not white. Another cause of the young lying
wet is nest watering by the doe (see above); this is recognized by the
strong urine smell and by the presence of faecal pellets in the wool of
which the nest is composed.

Deaths among 3–5 week old rabbits

Pneumonia caused by the low virulent *Pasteurella multocida* can
occur from the tenth day on; it usually poses no problem in the
unweaned.

Under poor hygienic conditions coccidiosis can appear, even at
this young age. As soon as the young begin eating solid food, at
around 3 weeks, acute typhlitis can occur: enterotoxaemia is
probably the cause (see Chapter 16). Coli-diarrhoea is observed also
in this age group but the highly virulent 015:H- strains cause more
problems in the broiler unit.

Raising motherless young

Whenever the doe dies before the young can eat solid food, at 2-3 weeks, a 'stepmother' is always the best solution. On industrial rabbitries the young are divided up among a number of smaller litters. Eight to ten kits per litter is ideal.
Note: one must be sure that the mother did not die from an infectious disease before spreading the young over the whole shed.

The age of the 'foster children' and the foster dam's own young should be as close as possible. In general this method is employed only during the first few days of life, although very calm does that are accustomed to frequent handling and nest checks will accept other young later, even when they are much younger than their own offspring.

When no foster doe is available, the following substitute milk formula can be tried:

homogenized whole milk	25 ml
coffee cream (18% butterfat)	75 ml
lyophilized skimmed milk powder	6 g

A vitamin preparation can also be added. 'Bottle-fed' rabbit kits should be fed 10 ml of this prepared milk only once or twice per day. In nature the young are also only suckled once per day. The use of a doll's baby bottle is recommended, or else a 10 ml pipette with a rubber bulb and a latex nipple.

The prognosis is rather bad, especially with newborns. Their intestinal flora does not develop properly, and death may even occur much later as a sequel to this: many such young die after several days from enterotoxaemia. Aspiration pneumonia is also a danger.

The substitute milk is administered by bottle or pipette up to the age of 3 weeks. From the age of 2 weeks on, hay, pellets and water should be made available.

Fertility problems

Infertility in the male rabbit

Congenital sterility, which occurs in a number of bucks, should be detected as early as possible by keeping good records of fertilization results.

Other causes of infertility include spirochaetosis (rare) and epididymitis and orchitis caused by *P. multocida*.

Infertility in the female rabbit

Some rabbitries have to deal with temporary or continual sterility problems in the does. The following is a summary of some of the possible causes.

Metritis (Plate 28)

Purulent metritis is caused, among other things, by *Staphylococcus aureus*, *Pasteurella multocida*, *Listeria monocytogenes*, *Salmonella* and *Actinomyces (Corynebacterium) pyogenes*. The first two occur frequently, the last three seldom. Another cause is the presence of one or more dead fetuses.

Metritis is usually only a matter of sporadic cases. Sometimes a sort of epidemic caused by *P. multocida* breaks out. There has been no research done as to whether this is due to strains which differ from those which cause snuffles and pneumonia. Another possibility is that one or more bucks may have epididymitis or orchitis, which are caused by *Pasteurella*. Upon mating they introduce these *Pasteurellae* directly into the uterus of the doe, which thereafter develops pyometra. This has to be tracked down by means of the rabbitry's record-keeping system.

Myxomatosis

Animals that have recovered from myxomatosis develop a temporary sterility which can last for up to 3 months. Vaccination, however, does not affect reproduction of does in large-scale rabbitries.

Prolonged interruptions in breeding rhythm

Breeding of does should be continuous. Industrial rabbitries employ an intensive or semi-intensive breeding rhythm: mating either postpartum or 10–14 days after giving birth. Fanciers breed does only after the previous nest is weaned. Does that are not regularly mated become fat and less cooperative in breeding.

Oestrus cycle

Rabbits are 'induced ovulators': mating triggers ovulation. Nevertheless does are not continuously ready to be fertilized: ripe follicles are not always present. It is supposed that the cycle lasts about 12 days, of which only 4 are infertile. Does with ripe follicles can be recognized by inspection of the vulva, which is dark red to purple; mating does with pale external sexual organs will result in poor fertilization percentages. During the less fertile period of the cycle, does are less willing to mate; when a doe does not let herself be mounted she should be brought back to the buck after a few days. If she still does not co-operate, the cause should be sought elsewhere. One should be aware of the fact that male and female rabbits, when placed together, usually do not mate immediately and that this part of his work always demands a lot of patience from the rabbit keeper. After a successful mating a buck shows a kind of spasm, and he falls sideways off the doe, sometimes squealing.

Anoestrus

There may also be periods of anoestrus, during the moulting season, for example. These periods of anoestrus often occur simultaneously among a large number of animals on a rabbitry, and often in the late summer or autumn. The initiating factors are insufficiently known and understood: light intensity, length of day and night, and temperature all play a role, probably along with certain ingredients in the feed. Windowless sheds with constant day and night periods and light intensity make for the least problems. The signs for this type of infertility are: refusal to be mounted, not becoming pregnant even after proper mating, neglect and poor nest quality with does that nevertheless do become pregnant.

    Treatment. Difficult since the cause is not well understood.

• There should always be a sufficient number of young does available to replace those that are no longer producing; this number is calculated on the replacement percentage.

• Sudden changes in light intensity and length of day and night can always be tried out.

• Placing the bucks in the vicinity of the does may help.

• 'Flushing' is also indicated, as long as the origin of the infertility is not obesity in the does. In this case, females should be rationed mercilessly until a few days before mating. Feeding *ad libitum* a few days before mating increases the number of ripe follicles. In the first weeks of pregnancy does can be rationed again, though less severely.

False pregnancy

In addition, the phenomenon called 'false pregnancy' can occur after unfruitful mating. This can also happen when several does, usually young, are housed together in one cage while being raised. These false pregnancies last about 16 days. At the end the doe often shows nesting behaviour. During the false pregnancy the doe will not let herself be mounted.

22 / Administration of medication

Methods of administration

Injections — technique

See Chapter 9

Oral administration

With larger groups this is almost always done via the drinking water. For various reasons, treatment via the feed is in fact better, but is only possible in very large rabbitries.

Rabbits are easily disturbed by an unusual taste in the drinking water. With 250 mg tetracycline per litre drinking water, the water consumption, and secondarily the feed consumption, can drop by 50%.

When greens or other feed containing moisture are given, whether or not in combination with pellets, drinking water consumption falls so low that efficient water medication becomes impossible. Instead, the medication can be spread over moistened bread or on the feed pellets. This method is often employed for the treatment of coccidiosis with sulphonamides. The dosage can be calculated per kg body weight, but it is impossible to know how much the animals have consumed individually when they are housed in groups. This also holds for treatment in the drinking water, but much more for the feed method because the medication is not evenly spread and because some animals eat more of a particular type of feed. A better solution is to delete the greens during the course of the treatment, although sudden changes in feed can also cause problems.

For individual treatment, oral administration using a syringe filled with suspensions or syrups is recommended. Paediatric preparations are often employed. The rabbit is picked up with the left hand by the skin of the neck and the ears, and held fast with the back down, under the left arm. The mouth opening is pointed upwards and the medication is introduced with a syringe via the corner of the mouth deep into the buccal cavity. When the rabbit starts swallowing, the liquid is introduced gently into the mouth. Help is necessary

in handling heavy or unmanageable rabbits. This is the easiest
method for treating pet rabbits, and also usually the cheapest.

Indirect toxicity of antibiotics

Some antibiotics produce high mortality in rabbits, and even more so
in certain rodents such as guinea-pigs and hamsters. Mortality rates
can approach 100%. Indirect antibiotic toxicity always expresses
itself in gastro-intestinal disorders. One to 14 days after receiving the
antibiotic the animals become listless, refuse to eat, lose weight,
develop diarrhoea and die; or, in rare cases, they recover. The
necropsy reveals a haemorrhagic inflamed caecum.

Many hypotheses have been brought forward to explain the possible origins of these disturbances. The most logical theory is that
after destruction of the normal flora, a resistant, harmful flora
develops. It has been determined that the cause is a toxin that is produced by one or another species of *Clostridium*. In rabbits it is
Clostridium spiroforme, in hamsters and hares it is *Clostridium
difficile*. How and why these bacteria, which are already present in
the intestines before the introduction of the antibiotic, suddenly start
multiplying is unknown. A spontaneous form of enterotoxaemia
which is caused by the same *Clostridium* also occurs in rabbits (see
Chapter 16).

The toxic effect of some antibiotics often goes unrecognized
because death does not occur immediately but after a variable period
of severe sickness, which may last from a few days to up to 3 weeks. In
addition, for a given antibiotic the mortality rate is not always the
same. This is not surprising since the toxic effect is probably
dependent on the flora present in the intestine, which can vary
greatly from animal to animal and from one unit to another.

Toxic antibiotics

Lincomycin and clindamycin are very toxic. Even a small single
dose, administered orally or parenterally, can result in 100%
mortality.

Antibiotics from the penicillin group produce mortality of from
0–100%. Ampicillin in particular exhibits a high toxicity, usually
40–80%.

With macrolides (spiramycin, tylosin, erythromycin, oleando-mycin) the risks are especially great when administered orally.

Well-tolerated antibiotics

Chloramphenicol is generally well tolerated, but can cause a decrease in drinking water intake. With preparations of chloramphenicol injected intramuscularly, a local irritant effect must be taken into account.

Polymyxin can be administered orally or parenterally in doses of 20–50 iu per kg body weight.

Neomycin can be administered orally: 100–400 ppm in the feed. For the treatment of severe cases of coli-diarrhoea up to 1 g per litre drinking water can be prescribed.

Streptomycin can be injected; 50–100 mg per kg. With higher dosages, the usual streptomycin toxicity can appear.

Tetracyclines are the most commonly used antibiotics for rabbits. For dosages of 250–1000 mg per litre drinking water, no harmful effects have been reported yet. Nevertheless it does seem to have an unpleasant taste in the drinking water since even with lower dosages the water and, secondarily, the feed consumption both decline. There is no problem when it is administered via the pellets, even in high doses.

Dosages

Injectable products

Oxytetracycline. 100 mg per kg live weight can be given, but only preparations that produce little irritation should be used. According to data in the literature, this large dosage, administered subcutaneously, produces blood levels that can remain therapeutically active for 2–3 days. We may presume that a good effect could also be achieved through a daily dosage of 50 mg per kg.

Potentiated sulphonamides. Injectable preparations can be given in doses twice as large as those ordinarily used for larger domestic animals.

Ivermectin. For the treatment of ear mange, 0.4 mg per kg can be injected subcutaneously. Local treatment against ear mange (rinsing and disinfecting the pinnae) is unnecessary when ivermectin is used.

Table 22.1 Drinking water dosages per litre of some commonly used antibiotics

Antibacterial agent	Dose	Remarks
Tetracycline	250–500 mg/l	Drinking water consumption falls above 250 mg/ml
Furaltadone	100–200 mg/l	Probably negative influence on growth at higher dosages
Neomycin	200–800 mg/l	Only for intestinal infections. In particular, for coli-diarrhoea
Sulphadimidine	1 g/l	Often used against intestinal coccidiosis. Also active against bacterial infections
Dimetridazole	400–600 mg/l	Also active against anaerobes

Oral administration

For the treatment of individual rabbits (pets or show rabbits) certain products, in drop of syrup form and intended for both humans and animals, are very useful.

Chloramphenicol (Chloromycetin palmitate syrup, Parke-Davis & Co. Ltd.). 50 mg per kg, or 100 mg per kg for serious infections.

Doxycycline (Vibramycin syrup 10 mg per ml, Pfizer). 4 mg per kg, once per day.

Potentiated sulphonamides (Septrin syrup, Wellcome, or Bactrim syrup, Roche). 40 mg trimethoprim + 200 mg suphamethoxazole in 5 ml. 2½ ml twice daily for a medium-sized rabbit.

Alternatively, Tribrissen piglet suspension (Cooper Animal Health) could be used. 1 piglet dosage = 1.1 ml contains 10 mg trimethoprim and 50 mg sulphadiazine. A large rabbit can be given two dosages per day. For baby rabbits whose weight is lower than 200 g, 0.1 to 0.2 ml per day should be administered in a tuberculin syringe.

Griseofulvin tablets (Fulcin tablets, ICI). These can be pulverized and sprinkled over the feed, or administered in a suspension (25 mg per kg live weight per day).

Mebendazole (Telmin KH tablets, Janssen). These can be crushed and sprinkled over the feed. 1 tablet (100 mg mebendazole) mornings and 1 tablet evenings, for rabbits which weigh more than 2 kg.

Mebendazole (Telmin 10% granules, Janssen). Recommended for the treatment of small groups: 1 g mornings and 1 g evenings, for

Table 22.2 Approximative consumption of drinking water and feed per animal per day, for breeds intended for meat production*

Age	Weight (g)	Water consumption (ml)	Feed consumption (g)
6th week	920	133	84.5
7th week	1200	177	113
8th week	1510	220	140
9th week	1810	243	153
10th week	2070	258	161
11th week	2300	267	165
12th week	2510	276	168
Full-grown (not lactating)	4000	300	150-170 *

* Feed and water intake vary greatly during gestation, especially in the last phase (4th week).

rabbits of 2 kg and more.

Fenbendazole (Panacur 2.5%, Hoechst). The 2.5% suspension is recommended for treatment of large groups. Dosage: 1 ml per 5 kg live weight (5 mg fenbendazole per kg live weight).

For oral treatment via the drinking water the dosages are given in Table 22.1. It should be remembered that daily drinking water consumption per animal per day amounts to about 10% of its body weight, and feed consumption about 5%. These percentages are higher for newly weaned rabbits, and lower for full-grown animals.

Between the ages of 5 and 10 weeks the water consumption is about 140 ml per kg body weight with breeds intended for meat production. In the twelfth week this is 110 ml. A weaned broiler rabbit weighs between 700 g (5–6 weeks) and 2500 g (12 weeks) More detailed data are mentioned in Table 22.2.

A non-lactating full-grown rabbit (meat breed, average 4 kg) drinks daily around 75 ml per kg body weight. During lactation the average drinking water consumption varies from 100 ml per kg (first week) to 160 ml per kg (third week). Thereafter it diminishes very rapidly. The individual figures per doe vary greatly, and are mainly dependent on the number of young.

The particular products listed in Table 22.1 for administration via the drinking water can also be incorporated in the feed. In that case the dosage should be doubled. Feed treated in this way is especially useful for the prevention of digestive system disorders shortly after weaning; so-called weaner feeds are pellets to which antibiotics have been added and many rabbit raisers use them for preventive or curative purposes.

Griseofulvin cannot be administered via the drinking water. It is sometimes used for treating large groups via the feed, with dosages of 750 mg per kg feed. As already mentioned, this treatment is rather expensive.

For the treatment of oxyuriasis in large groups of rabbits fenbendazole can be incorporated in the feed (50 ppm for 2–6 weeks) or thiabendazole (0.1% for 3 months).

23 / Traumatology and surgical intervention: castration

Fractures of the lumbar vertebrae

See also Chapter 18.

This usually happens as a result of incorrect technique in holding or carrying a violently resistant animal, or from children playing with the rabbit. After the accident the rabbit immediately falls unconscious and goes stiff. After a short time it wakes up again, but with permanent paralysis of the hindquarters, in most cases accompanied with incontinence of the urine voiding and defaecation. This last symptom is important for differential diagnosis with other types of paralysis. For definite proof, radiography is indicated. Fractures of other spinal vertebrae are rare.

Fractures of the tibia

This type of fracture is very common with pet rabbits. Treatment is not simple and the prognosis is at best dubious in the case of an open fracture. External fixation produces disappointing results because the skin is so loose and the animals try to shake off a cast or any other bandage. The best method is still to stretch the leg backwards and fix it, even though the position is very unnatural. A collar placed around the neck will keep the animal from chewing the cast or bandage apart. In some cases the broken ends of the tibia grow spontaneously back together beside each other rather than end-to-end, which results in a shortening of the leg. The function, nevertheless, is fairly well restored. Internal fixation could be very useful, but is seldom justified because of the high cost.

Sore hocks

See Chapter 13.

Castration of the male

With normal, calm rabbits, in the author's opinion, no anaesthetic is needed for castration, but it may be used at the veterinary surgeon's discretion or the owner's request. The helper sits on a high stool and lays the rabbit on its back in his lap. With one hand he holds the rabbit fast by the skin of its back and with the other hand he spreads the hind legs so that the genitals are easily accessible. A rabbit held fast in this way is, as it were, hypnotized and offers no resistance.

The method for a right-handed person is as follows: After local disinfection, the testicle is held firmly in place under the skin with the thumb and forefinger of the left hand, otherwise it will retract into the abdominal cavity during the operation. With the right hand a 2-cm long incision is made in the skin of the scrotum and tunica, parallel with the longitudinal axis of the animal's body. The testis and the epididymis are manually loosened from the skin. This is the only step to which the animals react in any way; the rest of the procedure appears to be absolutely painless, as long as the restraining technique is correct. The seminal duct is tied off with catgut. To prevent slippage of the knot, a needle is passed through the duct; a single knot is tied on the one side, and then a triple knot on the other. The seminal duct is then severed somewhat distal from the ligature. The remaining end of the duct is placed back in the abdominal cavity. The incision can be closed with stitches, though this is not necessary.

24 / Anaesthesia and hypnosis

Since the general rules of anaesthesiology also apply here, the general physical condition of the rabbit must be checked. Look out especially for chronic respiratory illnesses since these are so common.

Premedication with atropine is often prescribed, though in view of the high number of rabbits (about 60%) which are serum atropinesterase positive, routine premedication with atropine may not be helpful.

Making the animal fast beforehand is less important than with other animal species. Because of caecotrophy, the stomach will not be empty, even when the animal is kept from food for several hours. On the other hand, rabbits seldom if ever vomit, even with anaesthesia.

General anaesthesia

Injection techniques

The rabbit is quite a difficult animal to anaesthetize with injectable agents. Analgesia is often not complete even when relatively high doses of the anaesthetic have been administered. But in general only simple surgical procedures are carried out since the costs of more complex ones would easily far exceed the value of the animal.

Non-barbiturates

DISSOCIATIVE ANAESTHESIA WITH KETAMINE HYDROCHLORIDE

Dosages vary with different practitioners and with different routes (i.m. or i.v.); for intravenous administration 20–30 mg/kg is prescribed.

Ketamine HCl alone is not an effective anaesthetic for rabbits. A tranquillizer should be given simultaneously or previously. The different methods described in the literature have had varying success:
- *Diazepam* (1–5 mg i.v. or 5 mg i.m.).
- *Promazine* (in the combination Ketaset Plus: 100 mg ketamine +

7.5 mg promazine/ml; dosage: 75 mg ketamine per kg i.m.).
• *Xylazine* (3 mg per kg i.v.) followed by ketamine (22 mg per kg i.m.).

In our laboratory we have often used the combination of ketamine (25–35 mg/kg i.m.) with xylazine (5 mg/kg i.m.), administered simultaneously in a mixed syringe. In about half of the animals analgesia is not complete, and adding ketamine does not help much in this respect. With this method we do not premedicate with atropine, nor do we make the animal fast beforehand. Recovery is always good. The combination is easy to administer and safe, but is only applicable for simple procedures (for example, castration without a trained helper or of nervous animals, thorough inspection of the mouth cavity, treatment of abscesses that are difficult to reach). The induction period is about 5–10 minutes. This anaesthetic is often not deep enough for more complex procedures such as abdominal surgery or surgery of the eyelids, or for painful procedures.

NEUROLEPTANALGESIA

Fentanyl-fluanisone (Hypnorm, Janssen). According to the manufacturer's instructions, Hypnorm should be given at a dosage of 0.5–1 ml i.m. Without premedication, however, surgical anaesthesia cannot be obtained. Both diazepam and midazolam (2 mg/kg i.m. or i.p.) give satisfactory results; they should be injected 5 minutes before the i.m. administration of 0.3 ml/kg Hypnorm. Surgical anaesthesia starts after 10 minutes; duration of anaesthesia is 60–120 minutes. When necessary the antidote nalorphine can be given (0.5–1 mg/kg).

Droperidol-fentanyl. The commercial preparations Thalamonal and Innovar vet consist of a mixture of 20 mg/ml droperidol and 0.4 mg/ml fentanyl. A dosage of 0.22 ml/kg i.m. is prescribed.

COMBINATION OF LOW DOSES OF FENTANYL-FLUANISONE AND
KETAMINE/XYLAZINE

Fentanyl-fluanisone is given as premedication (0.1 ml/kg i.m.) and followed 10 minutes later by an i.v. injection of a mixture of ketamine/xylazine (7 mg/kg; 1 mg/kg). This combination gives a good surgical anaesthesia for 40 minutes, which can be prolonged by further administrations of ketamine (8 mg/kg).

ANAESTHETIC STEROID COMBINATION:
ALPHAXALONE-ALPHADOLONE

Short-term anaesthesia can be obtained by i.v. administration of the anaesthetic steroid combination aphaxalone–alphadolone (12 mg/kg). Also with this method analgesia is incomplete and thus it is recommended only for superficial surgery. Higher dosages (12–40 mg/kg) can be given i.m. and will act longer though, again, with unsatisfactory results.

Barbiturates

The use of pentobarbitone is generally not advised because of the narrow margin of safety.

Inhalation anaesthesia

Whenever possible, inhalation anaesthesia is preferred to injectable agents for the more complicated surgical procedures. Endotracheal intubation is difficult, however, because of the small mouth opening. A laryngoscope should be used, though the tube may be placed without visual aid. The latter method, however, risks trauma to the larynx and consequent laryngeal swelling which may cause death through asphyxiation. One method for endotracheal intubation has been described recently. Ten minutes after induction of anaesthesia with Hypnorm (0.5 ml/kg), the head of the animal is hyperextended and the endotracheal tube (3.5 mm), which has been prepared with lignocaine spray, can be advanced through the mouth into the pharynx. When resistance at the level of the glottis is felt, the tube is only advanced during inspiration, with minimal force. Correct positioning of the tube should be confirmed, following which the position can be secured with tape. Surgical anaesthesia can be maintained with nitrous oxide, oxygen and enflurane (Ethrane). Some authors, however, feel that the use of nitrous oxide in rabbits should be discouraged because of their 'pseudo-ruminant' behaviour, which may cause gas accumulation in the caecum.

The use of a mask instead of intubation is generally considered to be safer. Induction can be done in a respiration chamber, when this is considered necessary. A nipple used for baby bottles, with the tip cut, can be useful as a mask. It can be fixed behind the auricles, with tape. The use of an open circuit is recommended and the total air flow should be about 2.5 to 3.0 l/min for a medium-weight rabbit. The administration may be interrupted.

Recovery

Both under anaesthesia and during recovery the body temperature must not be allowed to fall too much. The smaller the animal, the greater the risk of hypothermia.

Useful tips for all small animals:
• The field of operation easily becomes large, relative to the total surface area of the body. Since this field is the main source of heat loss, its area should be kept as small as possible.
• Disinfectant fluids to be used on the field of operation should be warmed to body temperature.
• The use of either infra-red or normal light bulbs can be helpful during recovery.

Local anaesthesia

For abdominal surgery, spinal anaesthesia is also a possibility. After disinfection of the skin, 20 mg of the anaesthetic compound mepivacaine, or 2 ml of a 0.5% solution of bupivacaine should be injected through the lumbar spinal interspace at a level one or two interspaces higher than the iliac crest. The needle should be held in a caudoventral position (30° angle). If the injection is not made at the indicated level but two interspaces higher, the rabbit will be paralysed permanently. It is not known if epidural anaesthesia is sufficiently safe for pet rabbits, but the method is mentioned here for sectio caesarea because it is the only way to keep the fetuses viable. It is also advisable to place the newborns in an oxygen box for a few hours, especially when the mother has had general anaesthesia. If this is not done, nearly all of them will die.

Hypnosis

The special method of restraining the rabbit for castration, already discussed in Chapter 23, produces in fact a form of hypnosis. The somnolent state achieved with this method can also be useful for other minor surgical procedures. Hypnosis does not work with nervous rabbits.

The technique is as follows: The rabbit is carefully held by the skin of the neck and laid on its back. The hind legs may or may not be fixed. The assistant holds the head fast and carefully stretches it. At that point one starts rubbing the rabbit's stomach gently with the hand and speaking softly in a monotone voice. As long as the hypnosis lasts, the breathing remains deeper and slower, and the eyes remain open with the pupils somewhat narrowed. Whenever the breathing rate increases, or the animal moves, the surgical procedure must be suspended and the hypnosis technique reapplied.

25 / Euthanasia

The neck blow technique, which is used for slaughtering, is a good, painless method for euthanasia of young rabbits. It is not recommended for pets, though, because the owners will usually find it objectionable. Furthermore, many veterinarians who have no experience with slaughtering rabbits will have an aversion to this method and if so, it is better that they do not use it. The neck blow technique is difficult, if not impossible, with older rabbits.

The rabbit is held by the skin of the back or by the loin, as caudally as possible, and it is struck with the blunt edge of the other hand, or with a blunt object, just behind the ears. Immediately afterwards, the hind legs kick violently as if they were running, though this is only a reflex and totally unconscious. After a short time these movements stop. The animal should be checked then, by palpation, to make sure that breathing and heartbeat have stopped.

Another method which is also used for slaughtering consists of dislocating the vertebrae of the neck and is rather difficult for the inexperienced.

Newborn and suckling rabbits can also be humanely killed by placing them in a closed beaker with a tuft of cotton soaked in chloroform. With animals older than 3 weeks, the excitation phase is too painful; often they squeal with fear. (Note: for guinea-pigs this method is applicable for both young and adult; no excitation phase is observed.)

The intravenous and intracardiac injection of T61 or barbiturates is a painless method and is most appreciated by the owners. The technique for intravenous injection is described in Chapter 9. From 0.5 to 3 ml of T61 are administered, depending on the size of the animal; individual differences in the necessary dosage exist also.

Intracardiac injection is preferable with very young rabbits or with rabbits that are in a state of shock. The assistant lays the rabbit on its right side with the back towards him. The hind legs are held fast with the left hand, the forelegs with the right; care should be taken that the left foreleg, which lies above, is stretched well forward.

The one who administers the injection palpates with the fingertips on the ribs, just above the breastbone. With young rabbits and with those that are not too fat the heartbeat is easily felt. Where it is most distinct, the injection is made. Whether or not the heart has been punctured is determined by aspiration. If only the lungs have been punctured death occurs a little more slowly.

26 / Zoonotic aspects

The rabbit plays only a minor role in the appearance of zoonoses.

Tularaemia

This does not occur in Western and Southern Europe, at least not with domestic rabbits. In areas where the disease is endemic among the wild hare or cottontail population, domestic *Oryctolagus* can be contaminated through insect bites.

Pasteurellosis

Infection from bite wounds is possible.

Rodentiosis

Yersinia pseudotuberculosis can infect humans but infections are extremely rare. *Yersinia enterocolitica*, a related species which is not found in rabbits, is much more frequent.

Listeriosis

Listeria monocytogenes occurs not only in the intestinal tract of numerous animal species, including humans, but is also common in nature. The role of the rabbit in its transmission is unknown, though very unlikely.

Salmonellosis

Quite rare in rabbits.

Dermatomycosis

This is probably the only infection of rabbits that easily transmits to humans. Since this is also the case with almost all mammals, there is no need to go further into it here.

Toxoplasmosis

Rabbits are susceptible to toxoplasmosis, but while alive they do not infect other animal species.

Ectoparasites

Fleas do not occur in domestic rabbits, unless these rabbits run free and have contact with their wild relatives. With wild *Oryctolagus*, the rabbit flea is general. Rabbit fleas also bite humans. Wild rabbits that are heavily infected with myxomatosis and that let themselves be captured easily often turn out to be severely infested with fleas.

Cheyletiella parasitovorax

This is one of the common fur mites. It can cause a short-term dermatitis in humans.

Bibliography and further reading

Carman, J.R. & Evans, R.E. (1984) Experimental and spontaneous clostridial enteropathies of laboratory and free living lagomorphs. *Laboratory Animal Science* **34**: 443–52.

Catchpole, J. & Norton, C.C. (1979) The species of Eimeria in rabbits for meat production in Britain. *Parasitology* **79**: 249–57.

Clark J.D., Jain, A.V., Hatch, R.C. & Mahaffey, E.A. (1980) Experimentally induced chronic aflatoxicosis in rabbits. *American Journal of Veterinary Research* **41**: 1841–5.

DiGiacomo, R.F., Ralburt, C.D., Lukehart, S.A., Baker-Zander, S.A. & Condon, J. (1983) *Treponema paraluis-cuniculi* infection in a commercial rabbitry: epidemiology and serodiagnosis. *Laboratory Animal Science* **33**: 562–6.

Düwel, D. & Brech, K. (1981) Control of oxyuriasis in rabbits by fenbendazole. *Laboratory Animals* **15**: 101–5.

Flecknell, P.A. (1987) Laboratory mammal anaesthesia — long term anaesthesia using injectable agents. *Journal of the Association of Veterinary Anaesthetists* **14**: 111–18.

Fries, A.S. (1981) *Tyzzer's disease and the importance of inapparent infection in biomedical research.* Doctoral Thesis, The Royal Veterinary and Agricultural University, Copenhagen.

Gouet, Ph. & Fonty, G. (1979) Changes in the digestive microflora of holoxenic rabbits from birth until adulthood. *Annales de Biologie Animale et de Biochémie et Biophysique* **19**: 553–66.

Hall, L.W. & Clark, K.W. (1983) Anaesthesia in birds, laboratory animals and wild animals. In: L.W. Hall & K.W. Clark (Eds) *Veterinary Anaesthesia*, 8th edn., pp. 355–66. Ballière Tindall, London.

Hinton, M. (1981) Kidney disease in the rabbit: a histological survey. *Laboratory Animals* **15**: 263–5.

Hughes, J.E., Chapman, W.L. & Prasse, K.W. (1981) Cystic mammary disease in a rabbit. *Journal of the American Veterinary Medical Association*, **178**: 138–9.

Jones, R.T. (1975) Normal values for some biochemical constituents in rabbits. *Laboratory Animals* **9**: 143–7.

Kero, P., Thomasson, B. & Soppi, A.M. (1981) Spinal anaesthesia in the rabbit. *Laboratory Animals* **15**: 347–8.

Koosaka, S. (1974) Studies on gram-negative anaerobic rods in the fecal flora of animals. II. Distribution of gram-negative anaerobic rods in feces of rabbits and mice. *Japanese Journal of Veterinary Science and Biology* **36**: 231–6.

Laffoley, B. (1985) Chez le lapin les ingères alimentaires journaliers exprimés par rapport à l'unité de poids. *Bulletin de la Société Vétérinaire Pratique de France,* **69**: 117-34.

Lang, J. (1981) The nutrition of the commercial rabbit. Part 1. Physiology, digestibility and nutrient requirements. *Nutrition Abstracts and Reviews — Series B* **51**: 197-225.

Lang, J. (1981) The nutrition of the commercial rabbit. Part 2. Feeding and general aspects of nutrition. *Nutrition Abstracts and Reviews — Series B* **51**: 287-302.

Laplace, J.P. (1978) Le transit digestif chez les monogastriques. III. Comportement (prise de nourriture—caecotrophie), motricité et transit digestifs, et pathogénie des diarrhées chez le lapin. *Annales de Zootechnie* **27**: 225-65.

Mailhac, J.M., Demontoy, M.C. & Bomsel-Helmreich, O. (1980) L'anaesthésie générale du lapin domestique. *Receuil de Médecine Vétérinaire* **156**: 353-9.

Mews, A.R., Ritchie, J.S.D., Romero-Mercado, C.H. & Scott, G.R. (1972) Detection of oral papillomatosis in a British rabbit colony. *Laboratory Animals* **6**: 141-5.

Okerman, L. (1987) Enteric infections caused by non-enterotoxigenic *Escherichia coli* in animals: occurrence and pathogenicity mechanisms. A review. *Veterinary Microbiology* **14**: 33-46.

Okerman, L., Devriese, L. & Spanoghe, L. (1982) Indirecte toxiciteit van antibiotica voor konijnen, cavia's en hamsters. *Vlaams Diergeneeskundig Tijdschrift* **51**: 110-14.

Okerman, L., Devriese, L.A., Maertens, L., Okerman, F. & Godard, C. (1984) Cutaneous staphylococcosis in rabbits. *Veterinary Record* **114**: 313-15.

Peeters, J., Geeroms, R., Molderez, J. & Halen, P. (1982) Activity of Clopidol/Methylbenzoquate, Robenidine and Salinomycine against hepatic coccidiosis in rabbits. *Zentralblatt für Veterinärmedizin B.* **29**: 207-18.

Peeters, J.E., Pohl, P. & Charlier, G. (1984). Infectious agents associated with diarrhoea in commercial rabbits: a field study. *Annales de Recherches Vétérinaires.* **15**: 24-29.

Petric, M., Middleton, P.J., Grant, C., Tam, J.S. & Hewitt, C.M. (1978) Lapine rotavirus: Preliminary studies on epizoology and transmission. *Canadian Journal of Comparative Medicine* **42**: 143-7.

Prescott, J.F. (1978) Intestinal disorders and diarrhoea in the rabbit. *The Veterinary Bulletin* **48**: 475-9.

Regh, J.E., Lawton, G.W. & Pakes, S.P. (1979) *Cryptosporidium cuniculus* in the rabbit (*Oryctolagus cuniculus*). *Laboratory Animal Science* **29**: 656-60.

Spanoghe, L. (1984) *Etiologie en preventie van pasteurellose bij konijnen.*

Thesis, Faculty of Veterinary Medicine, Gent, Belgium.
Testoni, F.J. (1974) Enzootic renal nosematosis in laboratory rabbits. *Australian Veterinary Journal* **50**: 159–63.
Toofanian, F. & Targowski, S. (1983) Experimental production of rabbit mucoid enteritis. *American Journal of Veterinary Research* **44**: 705–8.
Van Cutsem, J., Van Gerven, F., Geerts, H. & Rochette, F. (1985) Treatment with Enilconazole spray of dermatophytosis in rabbit farms. *Mykosen* **28**: 400–7.
Van Kruiningen, H.J. & Williams, C.B. (1972) Mucoid enteritis of rabbits. *Veterinary Pathology* **9**: 53–77.
Wagner, J.L., Hackel, D.B. & Samsell, A.G. (1974) Spontaneous deaths in rabbits resulting from gastric trichobezoars. *Laboratory Animal Science* **24**: 826–30.
Westerhof, I. & Lumeij, J.T. (1987) Dental problems in rabbits, guinea pigs and chinchillas. *Tijdschrift voor Diergeneeskunde* **112**, suppl 1: 6S–10S.
Whitney, J.C. (1976) A review of non-specific enteritis in the rabbit. *Laboratory Animals* **10**: 209–21.
Whitney J.C., Blackmore, D.K., Townsend, G.H., Parkin, R.J., Hugh-Jones, M.E., Crossman, P.J., Graham-Marr, T., Rowland, A.C., Festing, M.F.W. & Krzysiak, D. (1976) Rabbit mortality survey. *Laboratory Animals* **10**: 203–7.
Yoda, H., Nakayama, K. & Nakagawa M. (1982) Experimental infection of *Bordetella bronchiseptica* to rabbits. *Experimental Animals* **31**: 113–18.

Further Reading

Cheeke, P.R., Patton, N.M., Lukefahr, S.D. & McNitt, J.I. (1985) *Rabbit Production,* 2nd edn. Interstate Printers & Publishers, Danville, Ill.
Harkness, J.E. & Wagner, J.E. (1977) *The Biology and Medicine of Rabbits and Rodents.* Lea & Febiger, Philadelphia.
Lebas, F., Coudert, P., Rouvier, R. & de Rochambeau, H. (1984) Le lapin — élevage et pathologie. Collection FAO: Production et Santé Animales. Rome.
Lockley, R.M. (1974) *The Private Life of the Rabbit.* Macmillan New York.
Marcato, P.S. & Rosmini, R. (1986) *Patologia del coniglio e delle lepre — Pathology of the Rabbit and Hare.* Società Editrice Esculapio, Bologna.
Portsmouth, J.I. (1962) *Commercial Rabbit Meat Production.* Iliffe Books, London.
Sandford, J.C. (1969) *The Domestic Rabbit,* 4th edn. Crosby Lockwood & Son, London.
Sheal, J. (1971) *Rabbits and their History.* David & Charles, Newton Abbot.
Weisbroth, S.H., Flatt, R.E. & Kraus, A.L. (1974) *The Biology of the Laboratory Rabbit.* Academic Press, New York & London.

Index

Abdomen, palpation 31
Abortion, causes 90
Abscesses 29–30, 54
  subcutaneous 40
Aflatoxins 16
Alarm signals 24
Alphaxolone-alphadolone 107
Anaesthesia
  general 105–8
  inhalation 107
  local 108
  recovery 108
Anal glands, abscesses 29
Angora rabbits 7, 18
Anoestrus 95–6
Antibiotics
  indirect toxicity of 98
  toxic 98–9
  well tolerated 99
Appendix, necropsy 34
Artificial insemination 21
Atropinesterase 16, 89

Bacillus piliformis 65
Bacteriological examination 39
Barbiturates 107, 110
Behaviour, pet rabbits 23–4
Bladder, diseases of 76–7
Blindness 31
Blood, drawing 27–8
Bordetella bronchiseptica infection 30
  respiratory 55–6
Breeding 21
  rhythm, interruptions 99
Breeds 5
Buphthalmia 51
Bupivacaine 108

Caecal impaction 71
Caecotrophy 13–14
Caecum, necropsy 34
Carbolfuchsine staining 38
Carcinoma, mammary gland 50
Castration 103–4
Central nervous disorders 31
Chest, necropsy 33
Cheyletiella parasitovorax 44, 113

Chloramphenicol 99, 100
Chloroform 110
Cleanliness 23
Clostridial enterotoxaemia 64–5
Clostridium, and antibiotics 98
Clostridium spiroforme 64
Coccidiosis 30, 31, 67–9
  intestinal 67–9
  liver 67
  paralysis 78
Coli-enteritis 30
Colon, necropsy 34–5
Conjunctivitis 30
  chronic 51
Constipation 71
Coryza 53–7
Cryptosporidiosis 70
Cryptosporidium 38
Cutaneous staphylococcosis 40–1
'Cystic disease' 50
Cysticercosis 70–1
Cysticercus pisiformis 70

Dental aberrations 86–7
Dental overgrowth 86–7
Dermanyssus gallinae 44
Dermatitis, moist 29
Dermatomycosis 29, 42–3, 112
Dewlap 9, 29
Diarrhoea 30
  Escherichia coli
    newborn and unweaned
      rabbits 60–1
    weaned rabbits 61–4
Digestive physiology 13
Digestive system 9–11
Digestive tract disorders
  aetiologies 58–9
  bacterial origin 59–64
Doxycycline 100
Droperidol-fentanyl 106
Duodenum, necropsy 33–4
Dyspnoea 30
Dystocia 31

Ear mange 29, 30, 43–4
Ectoparasites 113

Eimeria spp. 67–8
Encephalitis 79
Endotracheal intubation 107
Enteritis, viral 66
Enterotoxaemia 30
Enzootic pneumonia 53–7
Epilepsy 79
Escherichia coli 14
  digestive tract infection 59–60
  newborn and unweaned
    rabbits 60–1
  weaned rabbits 61–4
Euthanasia 110–11
Eyelid abnormalities 52

False pregnancy 96
Fasciola hepatica 70
Feed rationing 16
Feeding
  'backyard' and show rabbits 17
  in large-scale farms 15–16
  pet rabbits 17
Fenbendazole 101
Fentanyl-fluanisone 106
Fibre content of food 15–16
Fibromatosis 48
Flagellates 70
Fleas 44
Foreign body pneumonia 56–7
Francisella tularensis 84–5
Fur
  chewing 50
  mites 29, 44
  plucking 29

Genital tract, necropsy 35–6
Giardia 70
Glaucoma, hereditary 31, 51–2
Gram stainings 38
Graphidium strigosum 71
Griseofulvin 100, 102
Gut stasis 71

Haemorrhagic septicaemia 82–3
Hairballs 49
Handling rabbits 27–8
Hind limb paralysis 31
Histological examination 38
Housing 18–19
  and nesting behaviour 91
  pet rabbits 23–4
Hygiene 19–20

Hypnosis 108–9
Hypothermia 92

Ileum, necropsy 34
Incisors, malocclusion 86–7
Infertility
  female 94–6
  male 93–4
Injections 27–8
Intestinal coccidiosis 67–9
Intestinal disorders
  of unknown aetiology 71–3
  parasitic 67–71
Intestinal paresis in does 73
Intestinal samples, direct
  examination 37
Intoxications 16–17
Ivermectin 99

Jejunum, necropsy 33–4

Ketamine hydrochloride 105–6
Kidneys, diseases 76

Laboratory rabbits 7–8
Lice 44
Listeria monocytogenes 84
Listeriosis 84, 112
Listrophorus gibbus 44
Liver
  coccidiosis 67
  fluke 70
  necropsy 35
Lumbar vertebrae
  dislocated 78
  fractured 78, 103

Mammary gland carcinoma 50
Mandibular prognathism 86–7
Manure removal 19
Mastitis 40, 53–7
May–Grünwald–Giemsa
  stainings 37–8
Meat production 6–7
Mebendazole 100
Medication
  dosages 99–102
  oral administration 97–8
Mepivacaine 108
Metritis 53–7
  infertility 94

Middle ear
  infection 31
  necropsy 33
Milk substitute, formula 93
Mites 44
Moist dermatitis 29
Molars, malocclusion 87
Motherless young, raising 93
Mouth, necropsy 32
Mucoid enteropathy 71-3
Muscles 9
Myxomatosis 29, 30, 31, 44-8, 75
  cause 44-5
  diagnosis 45
  differential diagnosis 45-6
  epidemiology 45
  disinfection 46
  eyes 51
  infertility 94
  pneumonia 57
  prevention 46-8
  symptoms 45
  treatment 46

Neomycin 99
Neonates
  deaths among 90-2
  diseases affecting 92
Nephritis 76
Nest
  building 29
  watering 91, 92
Nesting behaviour, defective 90-1
Neuroleptanalgesia 106
Nose, necropsy 32-3
Nosema cuniculi 80
Nosemosis 31, 80

Oestrous cycle 95
Oral papillomatosis 74
Oryctolagus cuniculus 4
Otitis media 53-7
Ox eye 51
Oxytetracycline 99
Oxyuridae 71

Paralysis 78-9
Parasites, skin diseases caused
  by 43-4
Parasitic intestinal disorders 67-71
Passulurus ambiguus 71

Pasteurella multocida 31, 40, 51,
    53, 82
Pasteurellosis 30, 112
  acute 82-3
  chronic 53-7
Peritonitis 53-7, 74
Pet rabbits, behaviour 23-4
Pneumonia 30
  enzootic 53-7
  foreign body 56-7
Polymyxin 99
Pregnancy detection 21-2
Premature birth, causes 90
Pseudomonas aeruginosa 42
Pseudomonas infection 56
  skin 42
Pseudo-tumours 45
Psoroptes cuniculi 43
Purulent pleuropneumonia 53-7
Pyometra 29, 79

Rabbits
  functional uses 6-8
  history and taxonomy 4-5
  terminology 5-6
Rabbitries, hygiene 19-20
Rabies 79
Rhinitis 53-7
Rodentiosis 30, 74, 81, 112

Sacculus rotundus, necropsy 34
Salmonella typhimurium 81
Salmonellosis 74, 81-2, 112
Sinusitis 53-7
Skeleton 9-11
Skin diseases
  caused by parasites 43-4
  predominant traumatic 48-50
  viral 44-8
Skin
  infection 29
  necropsy 32
Snuffles 53-7
  cause 53
  lesions 54
  occurrence 53
  symptoms 53-4
  treatment 54-5
  vaccination 55
Sore hocks 30, 41, 48-9
Spinal column, necropsy 36
Spine, trauma 31
Spirochaetosis 42, 75-6
Splay leg 88

Spleen, necropsy   35
Staphylococcosis   29, 85
Staphylococcus aureus 40, 85
  respiratory infection 56
Stomach, necropsy   33
Streptococcus pneumoniae   42
Streptomycin   99
Sucklings, losses among   90–3
Sulphonamides, potentiated   99,
  100
Sylvilagus floridanus   48
Syphilis   75

T61   110
Taming rabbits   23
Tapeworms   70
Tetracyclines   99
Tibia, fractures   103
Torticollis   31, 79–80
Toxoplasma gondii   83
Toxoplasmosis   83–4, 113
Treponema cuniculi   75
Treponematosis   42, 75
Trichobezoars   30–1, 49
Trichophyton mentagrophytes   42
Trichostrongylids   71
Tularaemia   84–5, 112
Tumours   29–30

Tunnel digging   23
Tyzzer's disease   30, 65–6

Ulcerative pododermatitis   30, 41,
  48–9
Urinary system, necropsy   35
Urogenital system   11–12
Urolithiasis   30, 76

Viral enteritis   66
Viral skin diseases   44–8

Weight loss   30
Wool
  block   49
  production   7
  self-plucking   49–50
Wry neck   79–80

Xylazine   106

Yellow fat   88–9
Yersinia pseudotuberculosis   81